The Vulnerable Empowered Woman

Critical Issues in Health and Medicine

Edited by Rima D. Apple, University of Wisconsin–Madison, and Janet Golden, Rutgers University, Camden

Growing criticism of the U.S. health care system is coming from consumers, politicians, the media, activists, and health care professionals. Critical Issues in Health and Medicine is a collection of books that explores these contemporary dilemmas from a variety of perspectives, among them political, legal, historical, sociological, and comparative, with attention to crucial dimensions such as race, gender, ethnicity, sexuality, and culture.

For a list of titles in the series, see the last page of the book.

The Vulnerable Empowered Woman

Feminism, Postfeminism, and Women's Health

Tasha N. Dubriwny

Rutgers University Press

New Brunswick, New Jersey, and London

Library of Congress Cataloging-in-Publication Data

Dubriwny, Tasha N., 1976–
    The vulnerable/empowered woman : feminism, postfeminism, and women's health /
Tasha N. Dubriwny.
        p. cm. — (Critical issues in health and medicine)
    Includes bibliographical references and index.
    ISBN 978–0–8135–5401–3 (hardcover : alk. paper) — ISBN 978–0–8135–5400–6 (pbk. :
alk. paper) — ISBN 978–0–8135–5402–0 (e-book)
    1. Women—Health and hygiene. 2. Breast—Cancer. 3. Mastectomy. 4. Postpartum
depression. 5. Cervix uteri—Cancer—Vaccination. I. Title. II. Title: Vulnerable empowered
woman.
RA778.D865 2013
613'.04244—dc23   2011053240

A British Cataloging-in-Publication record for this book is available from the British Library.

Visit our website: http://rutgerspress.rutgers.edu

Manufactured in the United States of America

Contents

Acknowledgments   vii

Introduction: Public Discourse and the Representation
of the Vulnerable Empowered Woman   1

Chapter 1   Theorizing Postfeminist Health: Risk and the
Postfeminist Subject   13

Chapter 2   Genetic Risk: Prophylactic Mastectomies and the
Pursuit of Cancer-Free Life   33

Chapter 3   Postfeminist Risky Mothers and Postpartum Depression   69

Chapter 4   The Postfeminist Concession: Young Women, Sex, and
Paternalism   107

Chapter 5   Feminist Women's Health Activism in the Twenty-first
Century   143

Afterword: From Margin to Center   183

Notes   189

Bibliography   217

Index   231

Acknowledgments

Over the years I have been lucky to have an amazing support network of friends, colleagues, and mentors. While I take responsibility for any flaws in this book, I recognize that the book emerges from—and indeed my research process relies upon—the dozens of conversations, brainstorming sessions, hallway meetings, and chats over coffee with this group of supportive individuals.

Celeste Condit, Bonnie Dow, and Lisa Hogeland provided superb mentoring and advising while I was in graduate school. These three women stand as models of academic excellence, and I continued to hear their words of advice as I wrote this book. Kristan Poirot, Kristy Maddux, and Wendy Atkins-Sayre provided much-needed coffee breaks, laughter, and encouragement. For their open-door policies and willingness to answer questions pertaining to research and professionalization, many thanks to John Murphy, Kevin Barge, Randy Sumpter, Jim Aune, Barbara Sharf, Kathy Miller, and Leroy Dorsey. Marian Eide's keen eye and constructive criticism were instrumental in the writing of the book and in several grant applications. The members of the Writing Accountability Group deserve recognition for their thoughtful critiques of several chapters. I am in indebted to three undergraduates at Texas A&M who served as my research assistants from 2008 to 2011: Emily Heaton, Lauren Williams, and Michelle Ganoa. Many thanks as well to Luke Lockhart, who answered a last-minute call to help with editing. All of my colleagues in the Department of Communication and the Women's and Gender Studies Program at Texas A&M have been unfailingly warm and supportive.

Finally, I must acknowledge my family. My husband, Matt, stuck with me through the roller-coaster experience of writing this book. I could not ask for a more supportive and loving person in my life. My mother is the inspiration for this project, and my father is, in his own way, the instigator, for long ago he told me to simply "follow my bliss." My siblings have provided plenty of good cheer and good food. My "other mothers"—Aunt Vicki and Aunt Gail— are inspirations to me every day. Thank you all.

This project was supported with a Program to Enhance Scholarly and Creative Activities grant from Texas A&M University, a Faculty Stipendiary Fellowship, a Travel to Archives grant, and a Publication Support grant from the Melbern G. Glasscock Center for Humanities Research at Texas A&M University.

The Vulnerable Empowered Woman

Introduction

Public Discourse and the Representation of the Vulnerable Empowered Woman

In September 2009, the "Go Red for Women" campaign, sponsored by the American Heart Association, aired an hour-long prime-time event on national television. The show, "Go Red for Women Presents: Choose to Live," varied little from the "Go Red" campaign's main message since its inception earlier in the decade: heart disease is not a man's disease; rather, it is the number-one killer of women. With scores of celebrity advocates and a trendy logo (the image of a flowing red dress), "Go Red" has succeeded in making heart disease a very visible women's health issue.[1] Indeed, "Go Red" has entered the women's health marketplace at a time when many women's health issues are receiving more attention—from medical researchers, the lay public, and the media—than they ever have before.

The increased visibility of women's health has not gone unnoticed by the public or by scholars. Writing for the *New York Times*, Roni Rabin notes, "In recent years, women's health has been a national priority."[2] The flip side of this attention to women's health is, according to Rabin, a lack of attention to men's health. In what she depicts as a zero-sum game of health advocacy and medical research, the success of women's health advocacy groups in generating media and medical interest in women's health issues has led to men's health getting short shrift. The perceived necessity for advocacy for men's health is a remarkable, if ironic, turn of events given the state of medical practice at the beginning of the women's health movement in the United States in the late 1960s. Faced with a male-dominated health care system with a clear androcentric bias in terms of both research and practice, activists participating in the emerging women's health movement hoped to disrupt much of what was taken for granted by the medical industry, including the positioning of men at the center of medical research.[3] The increased visibility of women's health today is in part due to the diligent work by activists that dramatically changed health care policy, practice, and research in the United States.

As just one of many campaigns that owes its existence to feminist women's health activists, the "Go Red" campaign exemplifies the primary focus of my project in *The Vulnerable Empowered Woman*: public discourse about women's health issues. On the surface the purpose and main themes of the "Go Red" campaign replicate some of the main tenets of the women's health movement. Underlying much of the discourse of the "Go Red" campaign, for example, is the theme of women's empowerment and agency, as women are encouraged to take action and form a sisterhood. One description of the campaign explains, "Go Red for Women celebrates the energy, passion, and power we have as women to band together to wipe out heart disease and stroke."[4] Nevertheless, despite these similarities, some striking differences also emerge regarding the themes of women's relationship to the medical industry, the role of the medical expert in the health care encounter, and the context of women's health. Most prominently, unlike the critical stance toward the medical industry encouraged by the women's health movement, the "Go Red" campaign prompts a near-unquestioning embracing of medical knowledge and technology. Women's questions about heart disease are answered by medical experts, visually represented on the web site as white middle-aged men. The promise of collective action is contradicted by an overall focus on the individual woman's responsibility to take care of her own health.

Like a growing number of feminist scholars, I wish to revitalize the role of a feminist perspective on women's health, as the perspective offered by the women's health movement has been lost or misconstrued by the public and by medical researchers.[5] However, the revitalization I attempt in this project does not begin on a celebratory note. While I acknowledge that the increased visibility of—and medical attention to—women's health issues is one success of the women's health movement, approaching this visibility uncritically would contradict the explicitly critical stance of that movement. As an important source of laypeople's knowledge about health and illness, popular mainstream texts such as blogs, memoirs, advertisements, and the news are pivotal in making meanings about health issues.[6] My concern with contemporary public discourse about women's health is that such representations offer narratives of health and illness and identities for women that are easily aligned with a postfeminist logic. I argue over the course of three case studies that postfeminist narratives about women's health in mainstream public discourse align with neoliberal understandings of health that depict health as both the responsibility and the obligation of individuals and consistently reify traditional gender roles for women. The need to understand constructions of gender as integrally related to constructions of race, class and sexuality is clear, as public discourse about women's health is focused on a narrow group of individuals: white, privileged women. Where women of color do appear in postfeminist narratives about women's health, they are often positioned either as others who are need of paternalistic supervision or as discursively constructed "white" subjects who can be aligned with dominant cultural values. Through the positioning of women as vulnerable empowered subjects, women's health issues are depoliticized at the same time that some women's lives (namely, the lives of women who are white, upper to middle class, and heterosexual) are constrained to a narrow sphere of domestic activity.

Analyzing Public Discourse: Identities and Narratives

For my purposes, studying public discourse about health includes taking seriously the idea that discourse (language and other symbolic systems we use to understand the world) matters, a relatively commonplace understanding among scholars of rhetoric and cultural studies and feminist scholars of health and science. At the simplest level, recognizing that discourse matters is a recognition of the complex relationship between discourse and reality. Women's health scholars Adele Clarke and Virginia Olesen attempt one explanation by breaking down the nature/culture binary: "Nature does not exist outside of culture. This does *not* mean that what we might call trees don't compose what we might call forests or that you would not likely die if you walked out of a twenty-first-story window. It *does* mean that trees and forests have distinctive historical, cultural, social, economic, and discursive meanings."[7] Their careful recognition of both the materiality of the world in which we live and the discursivity of that material world points directly to the importance of discourse analysis.

If the example of trees and forests seems frivolous, I would suggest that it is the very commonsense understanding of trees and forests that provides its power and longevity. Stuart Hall explains, "Ruling or dominant conceptions of the world do not directly prescribe the mental content of the illusions that supposedly fill the heads of the dominated classes. But the circle of dominant ideas *does* accumulate the symbolic power to map or classify the world for others; its classifications do acquire not only the constraining power of dominance over other modes of thought but also the initial authority of habit and instinct."[8] The authority of common sense applies to the pink ribbons of breast cancer as easily as it does to the tree/forest distinction. For feminist critics, analyzing discourse is useful because of the way it focuses our attention on the "processes by which sociocultural hegemony of dominant groups is achieved and contested."[9] If public discourse about women's health is taken for granted, we miss our opportunity to ask questions about what meanings are being made for women's health and what material consequences those meanings might have.

I understand public discourse about women's health as productive "meaning making" discourse that shapes our collective understanding of (and thus our collective response to) women's health issues. Often offered through the ethos of scientific authority and scientific objectivity, many of the messages we receive about women's health are all too easily accepted as truth. However, scientific truth is, like the constructed meanings for race and gender and numerous other taken-for-granted ideas, a "thing of this world: it is produced by virtue of multiple forms of constraint."[10] Even the most seemingly objective medical statement is rhetorical, and rhetorical texts "work to make some ideas, positions, and alternatives more attractive, accessible, and powerful to audiences than others."[11] The "Go Red" campaign, for example, constructs meanings for heart disease that have material implications on a number of levels. Decisions regarding research priorities, policy initiatives, budget allocations, and diagnoses will be made based on the preferred understanding of heart disease as "also a women's disease." In addition, one of the key ways discourse shapes our reality is through the construction of identities. Juanne Nancarrow Clarke, a sociologist who has written extensively on representations of cancer, argues that humans never experience disease outside of language. In Clarke's view, discourse constructs not only our understanding of any given health issue but also how we live with certain diseases.[12]

I approach the study of language and symbolic systems from within a narrative paradigm that understands humans as storytelling creatures. Walter Fisher explains, "The idea of human beings as storytellers indicates the generic form of all symbol composition; it holds that symbols are created and communicated ultimately as stories meant to give order to human experience and to induce others to dwell in them to establish ways of living in common, in communities in which there is sanction for the story that constitutes one's life."[13] Narratives are, to use Kenneth Burke's phrase, "equipment for living": they help humans make meaning and act on that meaning.[14] When I look at public discourse about women's health, I see narratives about women's health that not only depict a certain understanding of a given health issue but also construct, or articulate, specific identities for individuals depicted in the narrative.[15] For example, breast cancer narratives over the past two decades have done extensive work in changing the identity of women with breast cancer from that of a "patient" or "victim" to that of a breast cancer "survivor." Without a narrative of breast cancer survival—of walking for the cure and wearing pink, for example—the breast cancer survivor disappears. In this sense, "narratives 'make real' coherent subjects," for without the larger cultural storyline, without a purpose provided by a narrative, particular identities cease to exist.[16] Of course, the narrative of the breast cancer survivor is not the only possible narrative one could tell about breast cancer; women's experiences with breast cancer demonstrate that the experience of breast cancer is far more complex that what the public narratives about that disease would suggest.[17] Public narratives about health do not (indeed, cannot) capture all versions of a health situation; instead, much like a media frame, narratives make certain "aspects of a perceived reality . . . more salient in a communication text."[18]

My concern in this project can be broadly construed as a concern with representational politics, or a concern with how, why, and with what implications women's health issues and women are depicted in public discourse. I emphasize at this point my concern with representations because all of the narratives I analyze are about real women, including celebrities with whom my readers will be familiar. My critiques of the ways women are represented in the narratives are not critiques of the actual women themselves or the decisions they make in the context of their lives. Because some of the narratives I discuss emerge from self-representation—often in the form of memoirs or personal interviews—the line between an individual's experience and her reporting of the experience may seem negligible. However, while a memoir is a literary work examining real-life events, it is also, like an interview given on *Oprah* or a news item in a newspaper, a representation of events.[19] Further, whether the broad narratives I identify are constructed in memoirs or news reports, each form of text presents a linear story, one written to appeal to an audience and make sense to an audience. Each of these rhetorical texts exists in a context of language; hegemonic understandings of bodies, lives, health, and illness; and common social and cultural institutions. Thus, for example, I understand Jessica Queller's memoir about her prophylactic double mastectomy to be a representation of that experience, and my critique is directed toward the representational politics of her memoir—the story that develops, the images used, and the language that crafts a specific understanding of breast cancer.

The narratives about women's health in public discourse have material consequences precisely because we act in the world based on the perspectives and identities offered to us in the stories that make up our lives. Writing about breast cancer narratives, Judy Segal notes that such stories literally constitute an answer to the question "How shall one be ill?"[20] My understanding of the power of public narratives—and the identities that they provide us—centers on the way such narratives are one tool we as humans use to make sense of the world. As such, the narratives I analyze in this project are not deterministic, but they do provide an example of how to respond to a health issue and they certainly inform our decision making and the roles (or identities) we take on regarding health issues. The difference between "determine" and "inform" is significant, for while public narratives play a role in how we understand our lives, they coexist with a variety of sources of information, from family and friends to doctors and pharmacists. Patients generally play a more active role in their health care than they did in the past, and women grapple with and make active decisions based on the medical information they receive and seek out from physicians, pharmaceutical advertisements, health campaigns, health-related Internet web sites, and mainstream public discourse outside the health arena (such as celebrity gossip magazines and television dramas).[21] Andrea Press and Elizabeth Cole's study of audience reception of televised plots about abortion points to how representations are "active forces" in women's lives in that they "interact with the thoughts and actions of particular persons, sometimes contradicting and sometimes supporting their beliefs and experiences." Through these interactions—of women with media and of women with other women, their friends and family, and doctors and religious authorities—the depictions of abortion become "ideas (or ideologies) that are *lived.*"[22]

Because I focus on mainstream public health narratives (see my explanation below), I understand these narratives as functioning as part of larger cultural hegemonic processes about gender and health; the narratives produce meanings about health issues and identities, or subject positions, for women that are reflective of dominant interests. I say this to emphasize an important aspect of my understanding of women's potential interactions with the narratives I study: namely, that while I understand women to be active in their interpretations and uses of the narratives, to deny the power of such narratives in informing the shape and texture of women's lives would be to vastly underestimate the role of symbolic systems in crafting human reality. I am arguing in part that as participants in larger hegemonic processes, women's health narratives do not exist in a cultural vacuum. I demonstrate throughout this project that the meanings and identities constructed in such narratives complement, even reify, postfeminist and neoliberal expectations for human subjects. The location of such health narratives as part of larger postfeminist and neoliberal discourses suggests that women are encountering similar ideas—and similar identities—elsewhere (on makeover reality television shows, in "chick lit," and so forth). In sum, while postfeminist women's health narratives do not determine women's relationships to the medical industry or their own understanding of themselves, I understand them to be highly influential.

The Vulnerable Empowered Woman centers on three case studies of mainstream public discourse about women's health: breast cancer and the rising use of prophylactic mastectomies, the normalization of postpartum depression, and the controversy about mandating Gardasil, the cervical cancer vaccine. My choice of the case studies was based on two factors. First, because this project is focused on narratives about women's health constructed in public discourse broadly (not the narratives constructed within the medical sphere or by medical professionals), I focused on health topics that were the subject of substantial public discourse that was not limited to health campaigns sponsored by the government or by health organizations. This narrowed the field substantially, as many increasingly visible women's health issues are visible because of strategic health awareness campaigns. Second, to support the claim running through this project that we (the public) receive health information from a variety of sources, I chose health topics about which narratives were constructed in many dynamic, overlapping media: advertisements, television shows, memoirs, health news, entertainment news, political news, and blogs.

Using textual analysis, I explore a range of media texts in the following chapters. What joins these divergent sources of material is their function as mainstream sources of information about women's health issues. "Mainstream" is my shorthand for indicating that the pieces of discourse I have analyzed are widely available and are more often than not positioned to appeal to the general public or at the very least to a broad cross-section of the public. The fact that women of color are only minimally represented in the narratives I analyze is in part precisely because of the texts (and health topics) that make up the focus of this book: postfeminist women's health discourse focuses on white women, while (less visible) narratives that focus on women of color populate media that are targeted toward, for example, African American women.[23] In my analysis, I pay particular attention to two questions: what narratives are created about women's health and, through those narratives, what identities are being constructed for women? Michael Halliday suggests, "Narratives are interpretative, and in turn require interpretation."[24] As part of my interpretation of the narratives in public discourse, I seek to understand how the smaller narratives of individual news stories and memoirs cohere to create a larger narrative (what Ronald Bishop describes as a "meta-story") that, in turn, "functions as an argument to view and understand the world in a particular way."[25]

By casting my research net widely to include a variety of popular media and news texts, I expect that the narratives I have analyzed are representative of dominant or hegemonic understandings of women's health issues. As a critic, however, I do not lay claim to truth. Rather, I understand my work to be a species of argument, and thus, like the very texts I analyze, my criticism is fundamentally rhetorical.[26] The arguments I present in this book are the product of careful analysis, but they are also products of my own social location as a white, middle-class woman and of my education in both interdisciplinary women's studies and communication programs. I understand my criticism to be a form of advocacy, as one of the underlying purposes in critiquing representations of women's health is to ensure that the visibility of women's health issues corresponds with actual health care for women that is woman centered, that is based on the complexity and diversity of women's lived experiences, and that is ultimately beneficial for women.

The Vulnerable Empowered Woman

I argue in my analysis of narratives about women's health that the current narratives offer a distinctly different understanding of health (a postfeminist and neoliberal understanding) than the narratives produced through the feminist perspective of the women's health movement, which emphasized issues such as collective empowerment, autonomy, and a critical evaluation of the medical industry. The emergence of postfeminist and neoliberal narratives as the most visible narratives about women's health has resulted in a new identity for women entering the health marketplace: the vulnerable empowered woman. For example, my brief review of the "Go Red" campaign's web site suggests the development of a narrative that revolves around the actions of empowered women. Featuring women of diverse racial/ethnic backgrounds, body types, and age, the web site tells women "The choice is yours" and offers a list of choices such as "I choose to donate to research" and "I choose to move, not sit." Women become empowered through the act of choice, framed in terms of consumption of medical treatments, diagnostic tests, and products such as red dress pins.

The web site also encourages women to take an active part in their own risk management: "Your body and current state of health are as unique as you are. That's why it's so important for women to find realistic heart health goals with the help of their doctors, and to be aware of the lifestyle choices that can decrease the risk of heart disease." Women who take part in the "Go Red" campaign are held responsible for knowing their risk and then managing that risk, often through lifestyle changes. The empowered women of the "Go Red" campaign are thus always also vulnerable women. Their ability (indeed responsibility) to manage risk is an implicit recognition of the female body's frailty, the dangers of the female life cycle, and the perils associated with living the life of a contemporary woman. Women are urged to talk to their doctors or to take the "heart CheckUp" not to find out if they are at risk but rather to ascertain their level of risk.[27]

The vulnerable empowered woman I have briefly sketched here is one who appears to have some agency and power to shape her own life. She is, in more ways than one, a thoroughly postfeminist woman who, through her various practices of risk management and consumption, functions to support a variety of neoliberal power structures, ranging from reifying traditional gender roles to supporting certain research agendas over others. For example, the management of risk for heart disease is, for this particular campaign, about individual choices and not about social and cultural factors such as the power of the fast food industry or the sedentary habits encouraged by the massive television and video-gaming industries. The agency of the vulnerable empowered subject is thus shaped by the meanings crafted for heart disease by medical experts and, in this case, the "Go Red" campaign's focus on heart disease as the problem of individual women, not society.

I am not arguing that the "Go Red" campaign has not succeeded in bringing our attention to the very real problem of women and heart disease. What I am arguing, here and throughout the three case studies that make up this book, is that while women's health is indeed increasingly visible, its visibility comes at the cost of its potential political implications. Why, for example, did the public have the misconception that heart disease was only a "man's disease"? How might messages from the "Go Red" campaign such as "Stop Smoking!" and "Get Physically Active!" serve not only to encourage individuals to quit smoking and increase physical activity but also to move focus away from potentially more complicated social factors that are correlated with heart disease? What does it mean to be understood as—and to understand oneself as—a woman with heart disease? These questions (and their answers) are effectively erased from the "Go Red" campaign. By erasing some questions and focusing on others—indeed, by making some women visible and others invisible—the narrative about heart disease reduces a complex disease and women's relationship to that disease to an oversimplified account of empowerment through lifestyle changes.

The vulnerable empowered subject is expressed in different ways in relation to different health issues, but in all it is an identity that places responsibility (and the moral judgments that come with responsibility) for health solely on women's shoulders. For clarity, in the case studies I discuss the vulnerable empowered woman identity through three specific labels (such as the cancer/ risk-free woman of breast cancer discourse) that indicate the variations on the vulnerable empowered subject. In each case study, I italicize the labels the first time I use them to draw attention to their position as the subject of my analysis. I use these labels not with the expectation that the identities will be understood as determining lived women's responses to public narratives but rather to emphasize the differences between how the vulnerable empowered woman is constructed in (for example) breast cancer discourse as opposed to cervical cancer discourse. Ultimately, I understand postfeminist narratives of women's health as part of current discourses on health and risk that, as Ann Robertson notes, "contribute to the emergence of a particular form of subjectivity—that is, a particular way of thinking about, relating to and situating the self in terms of the broader social and political context within which the self is embodied."[28]

Overview of Chapters

The constitution of the vulnerable empowered subject occurs at the dynamic intersection of postfeminist discourses concerning gender, health, and risk, and it is to this intersection that I turn in chapter 1. My purpose in that chapter is to offer readers—particularly those unfamiliar with the women's health movement or the concept of postfeminism—a concise overview of the main theories and ideas that guide my analysis in the next few chapters. I first offer a discussion of the feminist perspective on women's health that was developed in the women's health movement. I place the development of the feminist perspective on women's health in the context of the era of medicalization and discuss briefly feminism's role in the more contemporary development of the inclusion-and-difference paradigm. I then turn to a discussion of postfeminism, emphasizing how a postfeminist sensibility encourages the development of self-reflexive and traditionally feminine identities for women. I conclude this chapter by considering postfeminism in relation to risk, as the reification of traditional gender roles often occurs in response to discussions of risk that offer women empowerment through responsibility.

In chapter 2, "Genetic Risk: Prophylactic Mastectomies and the Pursuit of Cancer-Free Life," I introduce my first case study, which analyzes the prophylactic mastectomy narratives of Christina Applegate and Jessica Queller. I open with a discussion of the context for the case study, the contested nature of breast cancer research, and the construction of genetic risk related to the BRCA1 and BRCA2 gene mutations. I argue that the prophylactic mastectomy narrative constructs a specific identity for women—the *cancer/risk-free woman*—that compels women to make the choice to undergo a prophylactic double mastectomy. This narrative situates women firmly within the breast cancer regime and the biomedical industrial complex, leaving little room to question the possible reasons behind the rising interest in prophylactic mastectomies.

In chapter 3, "Postfeminist Risky Mothers and Postpartum Depression," I turn to the subject of postpartum depression. I begin by charting the history of women's health activism around the issue of postpartum depression and the tension between feminist and medical understandings of depression. The medicalized understanding of postpartum depression is particularly important for the central argument of the chapter: that postpartum depression is normalized for a certain group of mothers. Through my analysis of two memoirs about postpartum depression, popular blogs about motherhood, and news coverage of postpartum depression, I argue that contemporary good mothering is configured through a postfeminist narrative of risky motherhood. In this narrative women are positioned as *risky mothers*, and postpartum depression is one of many risks the risky mother might face. The normalization of postpartum depression, however, works hand in hand with a method of empowerment—surveillance—that restricts all women's actions as mothers and potential mothers and with the demonization of women who fall outside of narrative of risky mothering, namely mothers who harm and/or kill their children.

In the fourth chapter, "The Postfeminist Concession: Young Women, Sex, and Paternalism," I analyze the interaction between two different narratives that emerged in public discourse about the controversy over the Gardasil vaccine mandate in 2007. After offering a brief discussion of two key aspects of the context in which the Gardasil vaccine debate emerged—the use of virgin/whore dichotomy to understand women with cervical cancer and the health disparities associated with cervical cancer—I move to an analysis of both the advertising campaigns for Gardasil and noncommercial discourse (largely news coverage) of the mandate controversy. In the end, I argue that the commercial and noncommercial discourse combine to articulate a unique variation on the vulnerable empowered woman. Adolescent girls are depicted as *at-risk/risky young women*, an identity that reflects both a postfeminist mode of empowerment (they can choose to be vaccinated) and a clearly patriarchal understanding of women's sexuality.

According to Tania Modleski, "a fully politicized feminist criticism has seldom been content to ascertain old meanings and . . . take the measure of already constituted subjectivities; it has aimed, rather, at bringing into being *new* meanings and *new* subjectivities."[29] In the final chapter, "Feminist Women's Health Activism in the Twenty-First Century," I begin to answer the question of what a twenty-first century feminist health politics might look like. Through an analysis of three contemporary examples of feminist health activism, I argue that a new feminist health politics should include attention to the activist potential of health advocacy and/or support organizations, an intersectional approach to health inequalities, and a continued engagement with the gendered politics of health. These three areas of focus respond directly to some of the problems of postfeminist women's health discourse. I conclude by suggesting that feminist health activists should work to counter the dominance of postfeminist narratives of women's health by offering new narratives of their own—with alternative subject positions for women—in mainstream public discourse.

Chapter 1

Theorizing Postfeminist Health

Risk and the Postfeminist Subject

One of my primary arguments throughout this book is that contemporary representations of women's health have been disarticulated from feminism and that this disarticulation has significant ramifications for women. In this chapter, I offer a brief discussion of the women's health movement and the activist feminist approach to women's health that developed through the activism, publications, and theorizing of some segments of movement. It is precisely a feminist politics like the activist feminist perspective that is missing from current discussions of women's health in mainstream public discourse. I also offer a theorization of the current status of women's health discourse, which I see as drawing from postfeminism rather than from feminism. Postfeminism has usurped the position of feminism, bringing with it a representation of women as highly gendered individuals who are empowered to choose among medical treatments, manage their future and current health by altering their lifestyles, and increase or play up their femininity by taking advantage of ever-expanding opportunities to modify their bodies and lifestyles. I focus on how a postfeminist sensibility governs discourse about women's health through a larger rhetoric of risk in which women are represented as part of an inherently at-risk group that must engage in a constant monitoring and management of risk.

Feminist Activism, Women's Health, and Transformations of Medicine

The development of allopathic medicine in the United States can be roughly divided into three stages. The first era, from 1890 to 1945, "centered not only on the professionalization and specialization of medicine and nursing but also on the creation of allied health professions, new medico-scientific, technological, and pharmaceutical interventions, and the elaboration of new social forms."[1] In the decades after World War II, the jurisdiction of medicine expanded dramatically. Adele Clarke and Janet Shim explain: "By conceptually redefining particular phenomena in medical terms, and thereby effacing them as *social* problems, medicine as an institution became understood as an important new agent of social control."[2] Clarke and colleagues label this second period the "medicalization era" and suggest that it ended around 1985. After that, the dramatic changes brought on by technoscience and biomedicine ushered in our current "biomedicalization era."[3] The work of feminist women's health activists I describe in this section occurs in the social context of the medicalization era, when patients were largely understood to be passive recipients of medical treatment; medical professionals controlled access to and the creation of specialized knowledge; physicians and other medical experts worked through a paradigm of definition, diagnosis, classification, and treatment; and human bodies were expected to adhere to a standard norm.[4]

Although medicine "has no essence"—it cannot be reduced to simple social control or the management of social problems—and the process of medicalization has "made us what we are," the processes that were prevalent during the medicalization era in the United States were not equally distributed among the population.[5] Nikolas Rose asserts, "Some people are more medically made up than others—women more than men, the wealthy differently than the poor, children more than adults, and, of course, differently in different countries and regions of the world."[6] For the many women involved in feminist women's health activism, which includes women in the women's health movement and the numerous women who participated in feminist groups that responded to, supplemented, or at times resisted the dominance of largely white women's groups, recognition of women's specific role in the history of medicalization was an important step in a larger move to understand the many ways that gender and sex bias affected medical practice. Steven Epstein argues that despite the ubiquitous claim that "the field of medicine has long presumed a 'male norm,'" the history of medicine in the United States points to a more telling, and problematic, attention to difference.[7] Western medical theorizing about differences between social groups and individuals "placed European men at the pinnacle" by explicitly studying women, racial minorities, and other underprivileged groups and interpreting differences between these groups and European men as evidence of European men's superior intellect and physiology.[8] Epstein explains that understandings of (and research on) female difference can be traced back to ancient Greece. By the eighteenth and nineteenth centuries, the focus on women's difference "tended to construe femaleness as almost inherently unhealthy and viewed women as essentially controlled by their reproductive organs."[9] The medicalization of women's bodies and lives produced specific understandings of women as frail and inferior. These understandings were thoroughly critiqued by women's health activists.[10]

Feminist women's health activists in the late 1960s through the early 1980s can be best understood as positioning themselves as critics of the medical industry. They problematized the medicalization of women's lives and critiqued the passive role women were often expected to play in relation to more active, expert physicians. Feminist criticism of the medical industry took many forms. Radical feminists, for example, offered a "thoroughgoing critique of patriarchal practices and assumptions," while liberal feminists included medicine in their larger push for the "mainstreaming of women within all branches of U.S. society."[11] Feminism comes in many shapes and forms, and in this project I use an open-ended definition of feminism that draws upon what these many perspectives have in common. Andrea O'Reilly, writing on "feminist mothers," offers this understanding of feminism's common goals: "Feminists are committed to challenging and transforming this gender inequity in all of its manifestations: cultural, economic, political, philosophical, social, ideological, sexual, and so forth. Also, most feminisms (including my own) seek to dismantle other hierarchical binary systems such as race (racism), sexuality (heterosexism), economics (classism), and ability (ableism)."[12] Anthropologist Sandra Morgen describes the women's health movement as a "revolution" that transformed health care.[13] This revolution would not have been possible without the many feminist perspectives that informed the women's health movement. For example, the women's health movement may be best remembered for its radical self-help activities, including providing abortions and demonstrating how to perform vaginal self-exams with a speculum and a mirror. However, radical feminist health activists were complemented by liberal feminist activists, and both groups were challenged to create more intersectional approaches to women's health by women of color. The revolution brought about by women's health movement activists included arguments against the radical mastectomy, questions about the safety of the birth control pill and other methods of contraception, a focus on sterilization abuse in underprivileged populations, attention to problems of access to basic medical services, and theorization about the intersections of poverty, geography, race, and health.[14]

Chronological narratives of the women's health movement often begin with the actions of women involved in women's liberation in the late 1960s. Sandra Morgen begins her account of the movement with the 1969 meeting of women who became the now-well-known Boston Women's Health Book Collective.[15] The foundational stories that make up the movement are, according to Morgen, the story of *Our Bodies, Ourselves*, the story of self-help gynecology, the story of the development of the "policy wing" of the movement (eventually embodied through the National Women's Health Network), and finally the story of abortion rights and the Jane organization.[16] The role of women of color activists, specifically African American women, is treated in many chronologies as an afterthought with a notation of the creation of the National Black Women's Health Project (NBWHP) in 1983. Although Morgen's account does not fall prey to this problem, she covers the health organizing by women of color in a chapter separate from the foundational stories of the women's health movement. The separation of women of color from the usual chronologies of the women's health movement overlooks both individual activists and many organizations, such as the National Welfare Rights Organization in Pittsburgh, that took up women's health issues (often reproductive issues) from a feminist perspective.[17]

Because of the problems of some chronological narratives regarding the participation of women of color in the women's health movement and because of my own interest in a perspective that many different groups shared, I focus the remainder of this section on three facets of a feminist perspective on women's health that together make up what I call an "activist feminist approach" to health: the politics of knowledge, self-determination, and contextualization. The first theme—the politics of knowledge—encompasses a range of beliefs about the production, distribution, and validation of knowledge. Nancy Tuana describes the women's health movement as an "epistemological movement," one dedicated not only to providing women with knowledge but also to creating new knowledge.[18] Issues having to do with access to medical knowledge spurred the creation of the Boston Women's Health Book Collective and was also a prime focus for Barbara Seaman's landmark book *The Doctor's Case Against the Pill*.[19] Women's health movement activists wanted medical knowledge in women's hands, but they also performed extensive critiques of the knowledge about women's bodies and lives created by the medical industry. As Anne Koedt's famous essay "The Myth of the Vaginal Orgasm" so eloquently demonstrated, what passed as medical knowledge was always based in culture and reflected dominant values about gender and sexuality.[20]

In addition to theorizing about the cultural situatedness of knowledge production and critiquing women's lack of access to medical knowledge, activists
offered a significant challenge to standard accounts of objective knowledge by
insisting on the validity and importance of their own experiences. Women's
experiences with the Pill, for example, were collected as anecdotes and provided important evidence for Seaman's argument. The development and practice of an experiential epistemology within the radical wing of the women's
liberation movement extended to the self-help arm of the women's health
movement. Michelle Murphy summarizes, "Experience, as conceived within
the women's self-help movement, provided a kind of evidence that was used to
critique science, especially biomedicine, by providing a different knowledge of
the world."[21] More broadly, experience provided one foundation for women of
color to critique women's health movement activists that worked from the viewpoint of white, middle-class women. As just one example, African American
feminist groups "forged a theoretical framework about 'simultaneous oppressions' and reproductive politics in the 1970s."[22] The framework of simultaneous
oppressions was based in part on the knowledge women of color formed from
their experiences. Loretta Ross, an activist who directed the National Organization for Women's (NOW) Women of Color Program and was also involved
with the NBWHP, remembers her experience of sterilization abuse as a moment
that made her ask "what the hell is going on here?": "It was the fact that for six
months, I'd been going to this joker and his misdiagnosis and maltreatment
ended in sterilization. That made me mad. But that's when I began reading
more and paying more attention to how many women were sterilized. . . . I
looked at my sister and my mother. . . . There were very few women who were
ovulating in my family by their thirties."[23] Her experience of mistreatment by a
physician, coupled with the experiences of her family and her community, produced the knowledge that sterilization was "much more widespread" than she
had previously thought. Such individual and familial experiences by women's
health activists thus not only challenged medical understandings of women's
lives and bodies but also shaped the women's health movement's production of
knowledge and theories about their own bodies and lives.

The second theme of the women's health movement was often closely
tied to women's ability (or inability) to access knowledge: self-determination.
What I understand as "self-determination" is actually two interrelated areas of
emphasis regarding agency. First, women's health activists crafted arguments
about their rights over their own bodies. These arguments—often made within
the context of reproductive politics—suggested that women's bodies were

women's property. The Chicago abortion network Jane is an excellent example of women literally taking their health care into their own hands. Second, women's health activists made arguments about self-determination that emphasized the importance of women's agency in making choices about their own health care. Toine Largo-Janssen explains: "The perception of wrongful medical interference with the female body formed a central issue. This theme later expanded within health care into the notion of autonomy, authority over one's life, issues that were also valid and particularly important at times when decisions had to be made about illness and health."[24] In her work on breast cancer, Rose Kushner decried the standard practice known as the "one-step procedure" in which women were sedated, their breasts were biopsied, and, if the biopsy was positive for cancer, they underwent mastectomies without ever being wakened from anesthesia. Kushner's exposé was instrumental in establishing practices of informed consent regarding breast cancer surgeries. She argued forcefully for a "two-step procedure" that gave women an active role in the choice of breast cancer treatment.[25]

Where Kushner advocated for women's right to be active in the medical encounter, self-determination as voiced by other activists expanded beyond the patient-physician relationship and took on relationships that were often far more personal: those between men and women. In her 1969 essay "The Pill: Genocide or Liberation," Toni Cade, an activist involved in both the women's liberation and Black Nationalism movements, confronted the difficult question of whether Black women should understand the Pill as an instrument of genocide or use it wisely to control their bodies and destinies. Cade describes her experience at one meeting of Black activists: "Finally, one tall, lean dude went into deep knee bends as he castigated the Sisters to throw away the pill and hop to the mattress and breed revolutionaries and mess up the man's genocidal programs."[26] Although Cade clearly states that she does not agree with the idea (offered by some women's rights groups) that the Pill "really liberates women," she argues convincingly that it—and women's control over their own reproduction—is essential to the success of both Black Nationalist and women's liberation movements. She argues that women's right to bodily self-determination includes access to the Pill, which gives them time to "focus on preparation of the self" instead of abandoning control of their lives to others.[27]

The final theme of an activist feminist approach to women's health is contextualization. In her review of the important ramifications of the women's health movement for medical science, Largo-Janssen suggests that women's health activists drew attention to the "psychosocial context" of illness. She writes, "The operative concept of illness needed to be redefined as a biomedical concept that acquires meaning within the context of individual lives and social circumstances."[28] By "contextualization of health and disease," I mean, like Largo-Janssen, to point to the various ways women's health activists emphasized not just biomedical understandings of health and disease but also the social context in which individuals were understood to be healthy or diseased. Early conversations among the members of the Boston Women's Health Book Collective point to the importance of social location in determining one's experience of health and illness. Recognizing its members' own privileged position, the collective explained that "poor women and non-white women have suffered far more from the kinds of misinformation and mistreatment that we are describing in this book."[29] The Black women's health movement was pivotal in the process of contextualization, as such activists pointed not only to the inherent racism (often through ignorance) of some women's health groups but also to the social contexts of race and class as important factors in any discussion of women's health. The need for such contextualization was clear in the reproductive rights movement, for example. Byllye Avery remembers, "We told them [white women in the abortion rights movement] it was unwise to just talk about abortion. We felt like a lot of [black] children were dying from infant mortality and a lot of other things that were not being talked about. We never [focused on] a single issue at all, but they didn't listen."[30] Although admittedly an imperfect effort, the women's health movement did attempt to place women's health in social and cultural contexts.

The three facets of the activist feminist approach to women's health—the politics of knowledge, self-determination, and contextualization—undergirded activities as varied as the 1969 abortion speak-out performed by the radical feminist group the Redstockings to the development in the early 1980s of women's health programs in universities across the country. Through these varied actions, the women's health movement laid the groundwork for significant changes in the U.S. healthcare industry. Steven Epstein declares, "The legacy of the feminist women's health movement, then, was a deep skepticism toward the mainstream medical profession, a critique of many of its characteristic practices (including the overuse of such procedures as hysterectomies and Cesarean sections), and a strong emphasis on women's personal autonomy and control over their bodies (reflected in the concern with reproductive rights, but also actualized through practices such as the pelvic self exam)."[31] One of the more pivotal changes wrought by the women's health movement was the movement of previously private (publicly invisible) health issues such as reproductive health and breast cancer to the public sphere. Goods and services related to women's health constitute a major segment of the medical marketplace today. The "Go Red" campaign's insistence on taking women's risk for heart disease seriously is but one example of advocacy for women's health that, without some of the changes wrought by the women's health movement, would not exist. However, "Go Red" is also an awareness movement that does not acknowledge any relationship to feminism and does not privilege an activist feminist approach to health, despite explicit claims for women's empowerment.

Anne K. Eckman's explanation for the minimization of an explicitly feminist approach begins with the concept of the "Yentl Syndrome." In Isaac Bashevis Singer's short story, Yentl (a young woman) must disguise herself as a man to study the Talmud.[32] In medical practice, the term "Yentl Syndrome" refers to the practice of positioning men and male bodies as the norm. Former NIH director Bernadine Healy coined the term "Yentl Syndrome" in 1990 to describe how a woman with coronary artery disease must present like a man to receive treatment.[33] She developed this concept against the backdrop of a sensational report issued on June 18, 1990, by the Government Accounting Office (GAO) detailing the NIH's failure to implement a series of protocols from the mid-1980s that were created to ensure attention to women's health. As just one example, the GAO report described a study of 22,000 participants that demonstrated aspirin's protective effect against cardiovascular disease but did not include a single woman.[34] With the exception of reproductive differences, under the Yentl syndrome women and men were treated the same to the extent that a study with no women participants was deemed as applicable to women's health.

Eckman describes the report as the "D-Day of women's health" because it precipitated a shift in the early 1990s in the medical community from understanding the difference between men and women's bodies as located primarily in reproductive organs to understanding the difference as located in the entirety of the body.[35] This shift implied that in order for health care to be equal for men and women, the sexes had to be understood as fundamentally different. In short order, new research studies appeared (such as the Women's Health Initiative at the National Institutes for Health), new curricula were designed around women's health, and the popular media expressed a newfound interest in women's health.[36] Although on the surface this move replicates the call by women's health activists to recognize that women were more than their reproductive organs, it nevertheless carried with it problematic implications. Specifically, the "new body" of women's health as articulated as a response to the Yentl syndrome developed primarily in the furor over women and heart disease and was, by and large, a depoliticized body that existed outside of any social context. Eckman explains: "The new view of a woman's body as equal and opposite a man's construes a woman . . . as possessing social, political, and economic power equal to that of the independent, income-earning man."[37] In relation to this new, purportedly equal female body, a feminist critique seemed at best out of place and at worst misguided and narrow, as the feminist women's health movement has too often been reduced in popular memory to issues of reproduction.[38]

The shift to understanding women's bodies as fundamentally different from men's and in need of separate but equal treatment reflects a larger change in the dynamics of western medicine in the late twentieth century: the emergence of what Steven Epstein describes as the inclusion-and-difference paradigm. According to Epstein, the women's health movement played an important role in launching a wave of medical reforms in part because "once women put forward their critiques, they opened up a space of possibility that others could occupy."[39] Although they had many different goals, by the mid-1980s advocacy groups representing numerous groups (e.g., racial and ethnic minorities, the elderly, children) and specific diseases (most notably HIV/AIDS and breast cancer) had formed to advocate for inclusion in medical research and treatment.[40] Reforms enacted through federal laws and guidelines encouraged (often mandated) a focus on "research inclusiveness and the measurement of difference."[41] The result of such reforms, the inclusion-and-difference paradigm, reflects two substantive goals: "the inclusion of members of various groups generally considered to have been underrepresented previously as subjects in clinical studies; and the measurement, within those studies, of differences across groups with regard to treatment effects, disease progression, or biological processes."[42] Like Eckman, Epstein notes the potential problems of the new focus on difference, including the concern that the new focus on identity and difference runs the risk of ignoring other ways health risks are distributed and emphasizing the biology of difference (thus reifying, for example, gender as an innate essence).[43]

If the women's health movement put women's health issues on the table, many of the theories and ideas of the movement are difficult to identify in the inclusion-and-difference paradigm. Notably, the rise of the inclusion-and-difference paradigm that Epstein outlines coincides with the third era of medicine in the west: the era of biomedicalization, which focuses in part on the transformation of identities and bodies. One aspect of the era of biomedicalization is the move away from a universalization of bodies, or the expectation that bodies might fit into a universal norm. As Adele Clarke and colleagues explain, "Technoscience is seen as providing the methods and resources through which differences of race/ethnicity, sex/gender, body habitus, age, and so on can be specified, measured, and their roots ascertained."[44] Eckman, Epstein, and theorists of biomedicalization such as Clarke agree that the practices and purview of medicine—from how we understand medical research to the intimate interactions between physicians and patients—have changed significantly since the mid-1980s, when the focus shifted to difference, inclusion, and niche marketing. The transformation of medicine over the past few decades has had specific and often problematic implications for women and their health. For example, as Eckman explains, because biological sex has been repositioned as a foundational truth, "important questions about the construction of sexual difference as a category of analysis within research" are not a significant part of the creation of new biomedical knowledge.[45] To the theories of biomedicalization and the inclusion-and-difference paradigm, I wish to add consideration of the rise of postfeminism as one significant reason why the medical focus on difference today seems to lack a connection to the ideas or even the organizations of the feminist women's health movement. Rather than an activist feminist approach to women's health, the issue is now largely approached from a postfeminist perspective.

Postfeminism, Neoliberalism, and Women's Health Activism

I began my introduction with a discussion of the "Go Red" campaign, a campaign that is shaped by both the diminishment of feminism and emergence of postfeminism. This transformation is difficult to recognize at first glance because of postfeminism's relationship to feminism. The term "postfeminism" has been used to describe a wide variety of phenomena, and it most often appears in lay discourse to refer literally to a moment after feminism, a cultural moment in which feminism is (thought to be) no longer needed. I approach postfeminism as it has been theorized by feminist media scholars and social theorists,[46] who present it as a more complex understanding of the backlash against feminism. Susan Faludi's concept of the backlash points to the concerted efforts of anti-feminist groups to challenge the achievements of feminism. Within a postfeminist logic, feminism is not merely reacted against or challenged but is taken into account and to some extent incorporated into hegemonic power structures. Postfeminist culture, as Yvonne Tasker and Diane Negra note, works to "incorporate, assume, or naturalize aspects of feminism."

Thus, it is not a simple reaction against feminism, but a use or cooptation of feminism in a depoliticized manner.[47]

According to Rosalind Gill, our current culture's postfeminist sensibility revolves around the following issues: the notion that femininity is a bodily property; the shift from objectification to subjectification; the emphasis upon self-surveillance, monitoring, and discipline; a focus upon individualism, choice and empowerment; the dominance of the makeover paradigm; a resurgence of the ideas of natural sexual difference; a marked sexualization of culture; and an emphasis on consumerism and the commodification of difference.[48] This list of characteristics of postfeminism points to some of the ways feminist theories of empowerment and self determination are transformed through a neoliberal emphasis on individuality and responsibility into a discourse that shifts women's focus and energies from culture to self. Much like neoliberalism, postfeminism produces subjects that are "self-governing citizens who are 'obliged to be free' and who regulate themselves without the need for overt forms of state control."[49] As Gill explains, "At the heart of both [neoliberalism and postfeminism] is the notion of the 'choice biography' and the contemporary injunction to render one's life knowable and meaningful through a narrative of free choice and autonomy, however constrained one actually might be."[50]

Working together, neoliberal and postfeminist discourses have resulted in a women's health marketplace that is dominated by concerns for the health of individuals. Within this paradigm, the focus on the individual, while not always problematic, too often displaces a focus on the social. My concern with neoliberal, postfeminist health advocacy (such as "Go Red") is that without a clear feminist perspective on women's health, advocacy for women's health is reduced to offering (limited) choices in treatment, fund-raising for research, and the marketing of cause-related products in the name of profit and cultural capital instead of in the name of women's well-being. More to the point, when women's health discourse is not constructed through a feminist perspective, what is often diminished is a specific understanding of equality premised on an understanding of oppression as interlocking across the boundaries of race, class and sex. Taking its place is a neoliberal equal opportunity or "choice equality" that denies the presence of gender hierarchies and material structures that make opportunity a distinctly unequal phenomenon. Broadly speaking, then, women's health is currently being discussed, researched, and publicized in a cultural context in which all individuals are increasingly held responsible for their own health and well-being; consumption has replaced political action; negotiating risks means taking responsibility for those very risks; and equality is applauded but economic policies continue to reify (and indeed enlarge) disparities in the economic, political, and health conditions of diverse groups.

Managing Risk: Traditional Womanhood and the Vulnerable Empowered Woman

The neoliberal context of women's health prompts a focus on the individual, but not just any individual. Because neoliberalism and postfeminism are joined in women's health discourse, the subjectivity that is constructed in that discourse has a very specific relationship to gender. Postfeminist narratives about women's health position women as vulnerable empowered subjects who are empowered in relation to specific risks, but this empowerment consistently returns women to the most traditional of gender roles: naïve daughters, passive wives, and nurturing mothers. To clarify postfeminism's relationship with traditional womanhood, I turn next to a discussion of Angela McRobbie's concept of the postfeminist masquerade. In the case studies that follow, I suggest that in narratives about women's health, expectations about performing traditional womanhood emerge in relation to the vulnerable empowered woman's mitigation of risk. For this reason, I conclude this chapter by reviewing a governmentality approach to the social construction of risk and its application to women's health discourse.

The Postfeminist Subject and the Reification of Hegemonic Gender Roles

It is no coincidence that postfeminism emerged in concert with the rise of neoliberalism, as the logic of postfeminism revolves around the economically independent woman (the consumer), a subject made possible through a neoliberal emphasis on individuality, the free market, and the consumer citizen. The characteristics of "individualism, assertiveness and ambition"—attached specifically to the figures of young women—advance the notion of neoliberal meritocracy.[51] However, they do even more than that: the postfeminist subject provides at least one essential pivot point for neoliberalism by restabilizing increasingly unstable gender hierarchies. Although the postfeminist subject lays claim to the same discourses of individualism, responsibility, and meritocracy as the neoliberal subject, it does so within a highly gendered context. The result is a postfeminist subject that cannot shed her gender; instead, gender—and indeed traditional femininity—are magnified. The clearest explanation for the process of magnification and reification comes from Angela McRobbie, who suggests that neoliberal culture offers postfeminist women (who are most often represented in popular culture as young women) a new sexual contract.

This new contract represents an adjustment, or a give and take, by hegemonic cultural forces. McRobbie explains the issue: "The Symbolic is faced with the problem of how to retain the dominance of phallocentrism when the logic of global capitalism is to loosen women from their prescribed roles and grant them degrees of economic independence."[52] The newly economically independent woman holds significant potential to upend traditional gender hierarchies, especially as women's place in the work force becomes a commonsense part of culture. Once women are detached from the private sphere, the traditional "man as breadwinner, woman as homemaker" dichotomy can no longer easily exist. The new sexual contract for women is, in a sense, a replacement of this dichotomy. It places both men and women in the public sphere but maintains traditional gender hierarchies through a focus on heterosexual desire. Women in this new deal are invited to recognize themselves as "privileged agents of change" with an increasing role in the new global economy.[53] This economic capacity—presented as newfound freedom and equality—comes, however, with an emphasis on traditional femininity in various other arenas of culture, including fashion and health and medicine.

The new deal reshapes gender roles through a renewed emphasis on required rituals of femininity and the intensification of heterosexual pleasures in a way that actually restabilizes many of the more traditional aspects of gender. These required rituals of femininity are the new "postfeminist masquerade," or a way that femininity becomes etched across the entire body. The masquerade is a "new form of gender power which reorchestrates the heterosexual matrix in order to secure, once again, the existence of patriarchal law and masculine hegemony, but this time by means of a kind of ironic, quasi-feminist staking out of a distance in the act of taking on the garb of femininity."[54] In the language of the masquerade, the postfeminist subject who chooses to wear pencil skirts and stiletto heels and engage in the consumption of hyperfemininity through the fashion and cosmetic industries is not entrapped by gender norms but is ironically playing with them. However, although this masquerade may appear to be self-knowing and ironic, it works to reestablish patriarchal power through the reification of traditional gender roles.

As one response to women's increased earning power under neoliberal systems, the renewed emphasis on fashion—and the construction of a postfeminist masquerade in which femininity is taken on with a wink and nudge—is a reorchestration of the heterosexual matrix and a reification of patriarchal power. Most tellingly, the postfeminist subject who participates in this system may be highly visible, but she is also silent. As McRobbie explains, "The new female subject is, despite her freedom, called upon to be silent, to withhold critique in order to count as a modern sophisticated girl. Indeed this withholding of critique is a condition of her freedom."[55] This silent visibility offers up a highly feminine visible woman as a subject whose willing participation in western neoliberal economic arrangements is necessary for the new global labor markets to function but whose silence—particularly on matters of gender and power—is equally necessary if heterosexual/patriarchal hegemony is to be maintained. When a critique of patriarchy is abandoned, what remains is a critique of the self. Focused not on external power structures but rather on internal or self-oriented issues, the postfeminist subject engages not in political battles but in a process of constructing an appropriate life biography that is all consuming. As McRobbie argues, "Patriarchal authority is subsumed within a regime of self-policing whose strict criteria form the benchmark against which women must endlessly and repeatedly measure themselves, from the earliest years right through to old age."[56] The reinvigoration of patriarchal authority thus occurs through a sleight of hand, a moment in which a passive, hyperfeminine, self-oriented, self-reflexive subject is seen as being urged not by patriarchy but by women themselves. This reshaping of gender inequities, which is masked as gender *equality* through the language of choice, freedom, and empowerment, is a pivotal part of global neoliberal restructuring.

The postfeminist subject is a central aspect of my analysis of women's health discourse, as the arena of health is widely recognized as one of the places where the idea of "self as project" takes root. The vulnerable empowered woman's entrenchment within traditional discourses of femininity—including those about both behavior and appearance—has specific implications for the representation of breast cancer, cervical cancer, and postpartum disorders. In each of the case studies below, I explore the ways that dimensions of traditional womanhood tether women to one path of womanhood, from daughter to wife and mother. By "traditional womanhood," I mean a constellation of expectations regarding women's roles, behavior, and appearance that are derived from a patriarchal understanding of women as nurturing, passive, and pious. As subjects who make choices, women are represented in discourse about their health as free to construct their own lives, to take responsibility for their bodies, and to craft better selves. However, their choices are not limitless; their choices are shaped by highly gendered expectations for womanhood, prevailing market forces, and (in the United States) a health care system in which over 40 million individuals are uninsured.[57] Such choices are never free. Thus, the vulnerable empowered subject is a specific version of the postfeminist subject; that is, the vulnerable empowered subject is the postfeminist subject that emerges in health discourse. The key distinguishing characteristic of the vulnerable empowered subject is her relationship to risk.

The Social Construction of Risk

I have described the postfeminist subject as one engaged in projects of self-reflexivity and self-management, as a subject that is "subject to" increasing discourses of individualization and responsibility. Much of women's self-management and development regarding health emerges in response to larger constructions of risk that play a central disciplinary and regulatory role. Indeed, one way in which the self-reflexive postfeminist subject of women's health discourse supports neoliberal economic and cultural policies is through constructions of risk that downplay structural factors of health and play up the importance of traditional womanhood. In this sense, the inequalities clearly present in the health care system of the United States (research on privatized managed care, for example, demonstrates that individuals in poor health, low-income earners, and minorities report barriers to access and low quality of care) take a back seat to an individual's ability to manage his or her life and mitigate all possible health risks.[58]

I understand risk through a governmentality perspective that draws from the work of Michel Foucault in which risk becomes a practice, technique, or rationality through which governing is accomplished and authority is exercised. Mitchell Dean argues that there is "no such thing as risk in reality"—rather, risk is best understood as a set of ways of ordering reality, of "representing a set of events so they might be made governable in particular ways, with particular techniques, and for particular goals."[59] Critiquing risk is a multilayered project, for understanding how some issues/events/people become understood as risks/risky/at-risk and the effects of those understandings is what is important, rather than an attempt to objectively identify "true" risk. Dean writes, "It is important to analyse four dimensions of the government of risk. First, how we come to know about and act upon different conceptions of risk, i.e. the specific forms of risk rationality. Second, how such conceptions are linked to particular practices and technologies. Third, how such practices and technologies give rise to new forms of social and political identity. Fourth, how such rationalities, technologies, and identities become latched onto different political programmes and social imaginaries that invest them with a specific ethos."[60] I would emphasize the emergence of identities or modes of subjectivity in relation to specific ways of understanding risk. The role of self-management and the construction of one's identity in relation to risk is pivotal to the governmentality perspective. From a Foucauldian perspective, the individualization of risk leads to a form of governing in which individuals self-regulate. Responsible self-regulation, or discipline, is based on the construction of identities in which not taking appropriate action in regard to risk (or even not recognizing risk) is not a possibility.

The logic of risk assessment and risk identification governs contemporary health policy, and risk in public health discourse is often understood as the result of lifestyle choices individuals make. This lifestyle logic of risk encourages the development of public health policies that seek to promote health by changing individual behaviors. In the arena of health promotion and prevention, experts—scientists, doctors, public health scholars—have crafted a body of knowledge that is primarily focused on identifying and then changing what are seen as unhealthy lifestyle behaviors. Examples of health promotion discourse abound, including First Lady Michelle Obama's "Let's Move" initiative designed to combat childhood obesity.[61] Prevention of disease is thus intimately connected to constructions of risk, as the regulation of bodies now occurs through calculating risk and constructing risk profiles. Health promotion and disease prevention strategists discuss issues such as identifying risk factors (including personal behaviors/lifestyles and biological predispositions), identifying population groups that are at risk, and creating interventions that are designed to reduce risk. The identification of risk comes with certain expectations about risk-avoiding behavior, although such expectations are always in flux as new data sets might prove activities once understood as healthy to be "risky" and vice versa.

Risk and Women's Health

Scholars working on the intersecting areas of women's health and risk have taken careful note of the role gender has played in the social construction of risk. Indeed, as Alan Peterson and Deborah Lupton argue, the issue of health-related risks plays out differently for women and men; different expectations are assigned to each sex based on gender roles constructed in culture. Inserting gender into their discussion of the healthy citizen, Peterson and Lupton note that the concept of citizenship often implies equality: equal access to opportunities and institutions, equal status, and reciprocal rights and obligations. However, women are configured as healthy citizens in a context in which traditional expectations regarding femininity, womanhood, and motherhood influence expectations about health. They write, "Women in Western societies have been principally represented as citizens in terms of their contribution to [the] bearing and raising of children and the care of husbands and family members. The woman as 'healthy' citizen, therefore, is understood as a resource for the reproduction and maintenance of other 'healthy' citizens."[62] Women are positioned as responsible for mitigating risks involving both their own health and the health of their family members. In addition, two other features of women as healthy citizens emerge as pivotal in contemporary women's health discourse: the cultural assumption that women are inherently (read: biologically) vulnerable to disease (that is, they are always high-risk subjects), and the construction of women as "contaminated" or as carriers of disease (thus, women are also subjects that place others at risk).

Although the figure of the hysterical woman, the woman controlled by her womb and related hormones, may be less influential now than it was during the Victorian era, the figure of the vulnerable female always already at risk for disease continues to populate both lay discourse about women's health and medical discourse. Women are seen as more prone to illness than men. Far too frequently, characteristics of illness are conflated with characteristics of femininity and womanhood, including dependency, passivity, and weakness.[63] The result of this positioning of women is their increased entrenchment in fields of medical surveillance. In a similar fashion, the understanding of women as potentially contaminating agents—a cultural construction with a long history that includes representations of women's bodies as leaky and grotesque— positions women as needing additional surveillance. For example, prostitutes are frequently the focus of HIV/AIDS activism, based on the assumption that prostitutes—and their bodies—are harborers of disease. The experience of being always at risk and always placing others at risk positions women in a very specific relationship to responsibility and risk. Peterson and Lupton write, "Women, therefore, are seen as more susceptible to ill health and as more likely sites of contamination of others than are men, and as a result are regarded as requiring greater surveillance and control, imposed both by authorities and through self-regulation. Throughout women's life spans they are encouraged to protect their own health not simply for their own interests but because of their responsibilities to others."[64] Research related to the construction of risk and women's health issues affirms the centrality of these three related factors (women's biological vulnerability, their potential to contaminate others, and their responsibility for others) to the development of expectations for women's behavior, often in terms of how women manage risk.

Deborah Lupton's analysis of the surveillance of women during pregnancy points to the ways the feminine healthy citizen is positioned as responsible

for both the emergence of and the mitigation of risks. Women's double responsibility for risk is a distinctly postfeminist maneuver: women are empowered
(i.e., offered the ability to make choices) and yet their very empowerment is
based on their own flaws as women. Pregnant women are currently increasingly watched, or placed within "complex discourses of surveillance" that
regulate their behavior in relation to discourses of risk.[65] This regulation can be
interpreted through a governmentality perspective on risk as an example of biopolitics, or one of the ways a neoliberal state disciplines citizens (in this case,
women) through discourses of normalization that encourage a high level of self-
regulation. Of course, pregnant women are not only enacting self-regulation but
are also increasingly regulated by social and governmental norms according to
which what women can eat, drink, and do while pregnant are being codified
into law. Importantly, for the pregnant woman, taking care of herself is not
represented as a responsibility to herself but as a responsibility to her fetus. As
Lupton argues, "Her body, therefore, is constructed as doubly at risk and she
is portrayed as doubly responsible, for two bodies. Her unborn child is typically represented in expert discourses as fragile, highly vulnerable, its development susceptible to numerous threats."[66] In both lay and medical discourse
about pregnancy, there is no such thing as a "no risk" pregnancy because of the
assumed vulnerability of the fetus and the representation of the pregnant body
itself as deviating from the norm, the unpregnant body.[67] Faced with numerous risks both to the self and fetus, the woman bears responsibility for creating
and maintaining a healthy pregnancy and the production of a normal infant.
Women are ultimately held responsible for the moments when pregnancies do
not end in the production of a "normal" infant. Lupton suggests that pregnancy
has been reconstructed in our culture as a perilous journey that requires constant vigilance by both the woman experiencing it and the society that is witnessing it.[68]

   What is particularly striking about women's responsibility for risk management on behalf of the fetus is the way the risks that arise are attributed to
women. That is, women are not merely responsible for mitigating risks; they are
also responsible for the very materialization of those risks. Eating a proper diet,
practicing proper food hygiene, attending prenatal checks, taking the appropriate vitamins, and so forth are all ways that women can either mitigate a risk (a
woman might be understood to be reducing her fetus's risk of future asthma by
not smoking) or craft a risky situation (a woman might be understood to place
her child at risk for diabetes by eating a diet high in sugar). The construction of
women as having a double responsibility regarding risk may be central to the

complex meaning-making that occurs in women's lives as they interact with medicine. Research on how women experience risk suggests that interpretations of risk (and thus actions regarding risk) vary widely and are influenced not only by discursive constructions of risk but also by gender, culture, and situated meanings.[69] Kelly Hannah-Moffat and Pat O'Malley note that "for those governing through health policies, objective risk appears as the inescapable focus, and yet for many people it is one thing among many, something with an emotional price tag and something that changes its meaning when imbricated with social and cultural experiences."[70] Women's lived experiences of risk are complex, and risk can be interpreted in a number of ways depending on their life circumstances. Jessica Polzer and Ann Robertson's work on how women begin to embody the risk of breast cancer, for example, refuses to conceptualize women as "passive recipients" of expert knowledge.[71] Instead, Polzer and Robertson suggest that research that analyzes women's interactions with risk information "illustrates that individuals do not translate statements about risk unproblematically, but actively interpret risk information in ways that have personal meaning."[72] Interpretations of risk, of course, always occur within a specific social and cultural environment. Thus, Ann Robertson concludes that women's embodiment of risk aligns them with neoliberal notions of individual autonomy, responsibility, and self-surveillance.[73]

In the case studies that I turn to in the next three chapters, women's health is clearly oriented around discussions of risk, and women's responsibility for (often) producing and (always) preventing risk is represented as extending across women's life cycle and into many areas of health. One highly problematic aspect of the narratives of risk in public discourse is the reduction of the nuances of women's experiences with health-related risks. Women's relationship with biomedical constructions of risk is complex. It offers women the promise of better health, but only through continual self-surveillance. Hannah-Moffat and O'Malley offer this interpretation of women's lives understood through risk: "We often participate willingly in these regimes of risk because they promise, and often deliver, greater safety and security. Yet we buy in at a cost: we allow much of our daily lives to be delimited by considerations of risk that take into account futures that are unlikely to happen to the average person."[74] Replacing this complexity—including the ways women's relationship to risk factors and the decisions they make about perceived risks are "entangled in the moral, gender, and material contexts of their [women's] lives"—is a relatively straightforward understanding of risk that focuses on women's gendered responsibility regarding the prevention of risk.[75] The many issues that inform women's health related decision making, from personal interpretations of risk, familial relationships, and access to medical treatment to the cultural meanings of health issues are too often reduced in the narratives to a drive to conform to hegemonic gender roles. Women are represented in postfeminist health narratives as being offered a significant amount of agency in discourses pertaining to health and risk. However, women are empowered to make only a limited number of choices (often the choice between one treatment and the next), and their empowerment rests on gendered assumptions about their roles as daughters, mothers, and wives. Women's choices are, in this sense, constructed through traditional gender roles because they are often empowered to protect their own health for the sake of others (their families, their children). The discourses of risk that surround women draw directly from a postfeminist logic and contribute to the crafting of a postfeminist healthy citizen.

Chapter 2

Genetic Risk

Prophylactic Mastectomies and the Pursuit of Cancer-Free Life

For the week of September 15, 2008, both *Time* and *Newsweek* published extensive articles about the war on cancer. Both articles argued that while Americans have been actively engaged in the war on cancer for almost four decades, the war is not even close to being won.[1] As the title of the *Newsweek* article declares, "We fought cancer . . . and cancer won."[2] The *Newsweek* and *Time* coverage suggests that cancer, now more than ever, is a constant part of public consciousness. Breast cancer stands out even within this coverage as being particularly visible: the *Newsweek* article, for example, mentions breast cancer in the first sentence, offers a special information box called "A portrait of breast cancer," outlines a history of the "War on Cancer" that begins in 1971 and includes twelve items referring to breast cancer out of a total of thirty-nine items (thus, breast cancer makes up almost 30 percent of the events deemed worthy of recording on the timeline), and is surrounded by four advertisements and public service announcements that mention or focus on breast cancer.

This chapter focuses in part on the media coverage of Christina Applegate's experience with breast cancer. Applegate, a well-known and popular actress, went public with her breast cancer story and her decision to have what the media termed a "double prophylactic mastectomy" at the age of thirty-seven in early 2008. The media blitz surrounding Applegate's breast cancer experience fits nicely into the dominant popular discourse on breast cancer that privileges the experiences of young, white women.[3] Julie Andsager and Andrea Powers suggest that young women's stories of breast cancer dominate the media because they are understood to be more dramatic than the story of breast cancer that affects the majority of the population (the development of breast cancer during the post-menopausal period).[4] The drama of such stories often revolves around issues of women's fertility and reproduction. Further, the Applegate coverage is part a proliferation of public discourse about prophylactic mastectomies, an intensification that is made possible by many factors, including the development and increasing use of genetic testing for BRCA1 and BRCA2 gene mutations and the completion of numerous studies arguing for the efficacy of prophylactic mastectomies.[5] Applegate's story as presented in the media thus exists alongside many women's stories, including that of Jessica Queller, a television writer who published a memoir in 2008 about her bilateral prophylactic mastectomy, that combined create a clear narrative about prophylactic mastectomies.

As the daughter of a mother who was diagnosed with breast cancer in 1998, who continues to hear every six months about her mother's most recent mammograms and meetings with oncologists, who has watched her mother laugh with good humor at "chemo brain" and the other lingering effects of chemotherapy and continue to struggle with the use of her left arm, I read the stories of women's prophylactic mastectomies with fascination, anger, concern, and admiration. I make note of this mix of emotions here because I know that, much like my experience as I read the texts that make up my analysis, the readers of this chapter will likely have their own reactions. Of the three case studies I approach in this project, the choice of prophylactic mastectomy is by far the most controversial. I do not offer a final word on the "rightness" or "wrongness" of that choice in this chapter. What I wish to emphasize instead is the complexity of prophylactic mastectomies, from the agonizing decision to have (or not have) the procedure to living a life in a body that is vulnerable (or no longer as vulnerable) to breast cancer. This complexity is erased in the public narrative about prophylactic mastectomies. I hope that my critique of the shape of the prophylactic mastectomy narrative—a narrative that is all too persuasive in its vivid recounting of the horrors of cancer—is understood as just that: a critique of the narrative, not of those who choose to have (or not to have) the procedure.

In the prophylactic mastectomy narrative, the preventive removal of women's breasts is framed as a compulsory choice based on postfeminist expectations about femininity, sexuality, and reproduction. Deborah Lupton explains the centrality of these issues for breast cancer patients: "Cancer is one of the most feared diseases in modern society, and breast cancer attacks women at the bodily site where notions of femininity intersect."[6] For the young women at the heart of this narrative, issues of sexuality and reproduction are heightened because of their age: young woman may still be thinking of having children or may have young children to take care of, both issues that deserve consideration when deciding one's medical path. Although the twin issues of sexuality and reproduction may seem to be the natural focus of a narrative about breast cancer, these areas of focus work to not only sustain a representation of women that aligns with hegemonic, traditional womanhood (heterosexual, pronatalist) but also to reify race and class differences among woman and reaffirm women's dependence on biomedicine. The prophylactic mastectomy narrative represents women (particularly young women) as always at risk subjects who are striving become *cancer/risk-free women*. This variation on the vulnerable empowered subject combines postfeminist discourses of empowerment with biomedical constructions of risk and stratifies the breast cancer experience into privileged and underprivileged groups. The absence of a feminist perspective on breast cancer generally in mainstream public discourse (including the prophylactic mastectomy narrative) results in a blindness to the contextual factors that relate to the decisions women make, such as issues of race and class, and a mostly unquestioning acceptance of the necessity for (and overall benefits of) women's close relationship with biomedicine.

The Development of Contemporary Breast Cancer Culture

Contemporary breast cancer culture has its roots in the late nineteenth and early twentieth centuries. The American Society for the Control of Cancer (ASCC; later the American Cancer Society) was founded in 1913 for the specific purpose of "educating the public at large in the absolute necessity of operative treatment at the earliest indication of cancerous growths."[7] The early detection "Do Not Delay" message (to use the title of one ASCC campaign) was significant because it reoriented public understandings of breast cancer by reinventing cancer as a localized disease that could be cured by surgery. This transformation was begun primarily by nineteenth-century surgeons (foremost among them William Halsted) who believed that if breast cancer was local (only in the breast), the removal of all breast tissue represented a cure. Maren Klawiter notes that the diffusion of this view of breast cancer—one that necessitated a dramatic surgery for individual women—was dependent upon a variety of cultural and medical transformations, including the institutionalization of the Halsted radical mastectomy in American medicine, the standardization of medical education and practice, the growing use and efficacy of anesthetics, and the development of a passive, sick subjectivity for breast cancer patients.[8]

Klawiter describes the above configuration of breast cancer as the "regime of medicalization." This regime offered women a very specific understanding of breast cancer that focused on the efficacy of early detection as a preventive strategy, a passive role for women as patients, a focus on maintaining femininity and returning women to their normal lives after treatment, and the public invisibility of breast cancer. By "public invisibility," I do not mean to suggest that breast cancer was not discussed in the public sphere (women's magazines, for example, had long offered coverage of cancer that echoed the ASCC's early detection message). As Kirsten E. Gardner notes, "Historians need to cast a more critical eye on this concept of false modesty among women and cancer in the twentieth century. It is obvious that by midcentury large numbers of women had learned about cancer, discussed it among themselves, and organized to teach a broader audience."[9] What I mean to point to is the relative invisibility of breast cancer patients, both to each other and to the broader public. Klawiter explains that the role of mastectomees during this regime "required that, upon leaving the hospital, they return to their normal lives and hide the evidence of their surgery."[10] Groups such as Reach for Recovery aided in the invisibility of the breast cancer patient by stressing the importance of prostheses and promising women that with the right prosthesis and the right makeup, their breast cancer experience did not have to be public knowledge.

Through the 1970s and 1980s, medical knowledge of and medical practices regarding breast cancer shifted substantially. The Halsted radical mastectomy, for example, fell out of favor with surgeons who were finally convinced by the growing evidence that less-mutilating surgeries offered women similar survival periods. During this period, the "regime of medicalization" was supplanted by a "regime of biomedicalization," in which discourses of risk guided both treatment and the development of new breast cancer subjectivities. The role of the breast cancer patient changed significantly not because the early detection message of the previous regime had changed but because asymptomatic women were folded into the larger discourse on breast cancer as mammogram screening became widespread. During the previous regime, women had been told to look for danger signs because early detection could help doctors treat the disease successfully, but women who never found danger signs never entered the medical arena or took part in the culture of breast cancer. With the advent of routine mammogram screening, asymptomatic women became subjects "at risk" and were "reconstituted as permanent subjects of the disease regime."[11] This reshaping of subjectivities for breast cancer patients is part of what Adele Clarke and colleagues describe as the era of biomedicalization. Clarke and colleagues note the importance of identities and bodies to biomedicalization: "Opportunities for biomedicalization extend beyond merely regulating and controlling what bodies can (and cannot) or should (and should not) do to also focus on assessing, shifting, reconstituting, and ultimately transforming bodies for varying purposes, including new identities."[12]

Feminist health activism in the 1970s and 1980s also played a role in challenging (and changing) some of the basic tenets of existing breast cancer culture, including the need for passive patients, a reliance on invasive surgery, and a belief in the effectiveness of early detection. Feminist writers Rose Kushner and Audre Lorde decried the paternalistic treatment of women as breast cancer patients; Kushner's best-selling 1975 book *Breast Cancer: A Personal History and Investigative Report* presented a strong argument for the abandonment of the "one-step" procedure that often resulted in mastectomies at the same time as biopsies. Patients gained the right to "gaze back" at their physicians, ask questions, and become participants in their own treatment decisions. With this new gaze, women increasingly sought more information about breast cancer, and in the 1970s and 1980s cancer support groups emerged as pivotal sources of empowerment for women with cancer. Many of these groups were founded with or by women's rights activists, not unlike the development of postpartum depression self-help groups in the 1980s.[13] The role of support groups cannot be overstated; as Klawiter notes, support groups "made members of the breast cancer society visible to each other."[14] The concurrent development of breast cancer advocacy organizations (both grassroots and professional organizations) and biomedical advances made breast cancer patients visible to the world.

Professional breast cancer organizations (organizations that work for women's health equity and "do not identify either with broader movements for social change or with feminism per se") shifted the identity of breast cancer patients from individuals who were ill to a larger "collectively shared, publicly declared, political identity": the breast cancer survivor.[15] Perhaps the most visible breast cancer organization in the United States is Susan G. Komen for the Cure, founded in 1982 by Nancy Brinker (named in honor of her sister who died of breast cancer in 1980 at the age of thirty-six).[16] Komen for the Cure embraces the message of early detection through routine mammogram screening. Each year, hundreds of thousands of individuals participate the organization's "Race for the Cure," a major fund-raising event for the group. Although breast cancer activism takes many forms and grassroots organizations such as Breast Cancer Action (BCA) do offer alternatives, professional organizations dominate public discourse. Their dominance is significant because of how professional groups position women in relation to biomedicine. Professional groups have embraced the promise of biomedicine. Framing biomedical techniques as hope technologies, these groups join many individuals and scholars in hoping "that advances in biomedicine will alleviate suffering, avert much illness, lead to the development of more effective and safer drugs, allow the infertile to have children, cure conditions that are currently untreatable and much more."[17] Thus, Komen for the Cure encourages women to "race for the cure" because a cure is feasible, even probable, in the context of new biomedical technology.

Dominant breast cancer culture currently positions women as active (indeed, eager) consumers of biomedical advances, and breast cancer research reflects the concerns of the early detection advocates (early detection continues to be framed as prevention). Samantha King writes that mainstream discourse on the outcomes of breast cancer research "relies heavily—and often uncritically—on the language of 'progress,' 'breakthrough,' and 'cure,'" although it is unclear whether the high level of funding has positively affected breast cancer incidence and mortality rates.[18] The uncritical aspect of dominant breast cancer culture is particularly worrisome given the very contentious nature of breast cancer research. Given the many unknowns of breast cancer etiology, research on how to prevent and/or cure breast cancer has produced highly uncertain knowledge (although this uncertainty is perhaps not clearly understood by the lay public). For example, despite the always-contentious nature of radical mastectomies (as many of 75 percent of women who had received radical mastectomies eventually died of breast cancer, suggesting that the promise of a "cure" offered by the procedure was far from straightforward), ultimately the "focus on research oriented toward early detection and treatment (or 'cure') emerged in the late-nineteenth century and has remained the dominant mode of approaching the disease ever since."[19] Contemporary controversies over the "curative nature" of breast cancer treatments such as high-dose chemotherapy and bone-marrow transplants point to what Barron Lerner describes as the "enduring zeal with which American society approaches the possibility of a cure."[20]

The staying power of the discourse of early detection and cure was made clear most recently during the 2009 controversy regarding mammogram screening guidelines. As Jennifer Fosket notes, "Mammography and breast self-exam have maintained a stronghold while always remaining controversial."[21] In 2009, the U.S. Preventive Services Task Force issued a statement arguing that women in their forties should not be receiving routine screening. *New York Times* reporter Gina Kolata noted that this reversal of guidelines (seven years earlier the same group had recommended routine mammograms for women in their forties) would likely "touch off another round of controversy" regarding breast cancer detection, and she was correct.[22] The firestorm was immediate and women were among the stakeholders arguing both for and against the change. Many women expressed the desire to receive mammogram screening in their forties, while others (often associated with feminist activist groups) expressed approval of the new changes.[23] Some two years later, despite clear disagreements about the efficacy and safety of routine mammogram screening, the controversies about mammograms have once again disappeared. The ACS, for example, offers one simple statement on its web site: "Women age 40 and older should have a screening mammogram every year and should keep on doing so for as long as they are in good health. While mammograms can miss some cancers, they are still a very good way to find breast cancer."[24] The ACS is continuing a pattern Klawiter noted in her analysis of the screening controversies: "[The] message of uncertainty and ambiguity . . . continues to be rejected by the overwhelming majority of health providers and public health professionals."[25]

Genetics and the Construction of Risk in Dominant Breast Cancer Culture

Alan Peterson and Deborah Lupton suggest that within "contemporary Western societies the health status and vulnerability of the body are central themes of existence."[26] This is certainly true within dominant breast cancer culture populated by the construction of the breast cancer survivor. The push for individuals to take responsibility for their health and manage their relationship to risk is seen in survivor culture in the all-too-common discourse of individual risk factors for breast cancer and the widely touted lifetime risk of one in eight that a woman will have breast cancer. What has changed in terms of the discourse about breast cancer risk in the past two decades is the focus on genetics. After the discovery of the BRCA1 and BRCA2 genetic mutations, Myriad Genetic Laboratories developed and patented a commercially viable genetic screening test that was made available in 1998.[27] Myriad began heavily marketing its test directly to consumers, thus expanding the already-increasing numbers of risky subjects within breast cancer discourse.[28] Contemporary focus on genetics is a key aspect of the era of biomedicalization and what Rose calls "vital politics," or the politics of life itself. New constructions of genetic susceptibility differ significantly from previous constructions of hereditary susceptibility because within a "vital politics," taking action based on genetic susceptibility holds the "promise of a transformed, less-diseased future for individuals."[29] In this section I offer a critique of dominant breast cancer culture's constructions of "lifestyle" risks and unavoidable risks and suggest that this framing of risk prompts specific forms of surveillance and action, most notably a compulsion to prevent breast cancer through risk management.

Risk factors are contested biomedical terrain. According to Fosket, "Risk factors are mutable; they vary in importance and are supported by various degrees of evidence within social, economic, cultural, and political milieus."[30] The contested nature of risk, however, disappears in reports from mainstream cancer organizations of risk factors for breast cancer. The NCI and the ACS offer broad definitions of risk. For the ACS, a risk factor is "anything that affects a person's chance of getting a disease such as cancer," while the NCI describes risk factors as "something that increases the chance of developing a disease."[31] The NCI, the ACS and Komen for the Cure also demonstrate unity in their framing of categories of risk by delineating two categories that are based in a concept of individual control. Importantly, both categories of risk—risks that individuals have control over and risks that are out of individuals' control—are clearly linked to specific actions. In other words, even a risk that is out of control is "actionable." Komen for the Cure explains, "There are some risk factors you can control, and others you cannot."[32] However, "knowing the basic types of risk can help you understand your chances of getting breast cancer and the steps you can take to lower your risk."[33]

The NCI uses the language of avoidance to point to individual control of risk; thus, risks such as smoking are understood as "avoidable."[34] The ACS offers a list of controllable risk factors framed as "lifestyle choices," or things that the individual can change. In this list, issues such as smoking, using birth control pills, or imbibing alcohol all indicate a "higher risk" of breast cancer.[35] The avoidable risks that appear as lists on most breast cancer web sites are the product of long-standing scientific debates.[36] "Lifestyle" or "avoidable" risks as represented in mainstream cancer organizations are one clear depiction of how the burden for reducing one's risk of breast cancer is placed on individual women. Risk in this discourse is often tied with choice, reflecting the broader shift in health promotion strategies in neoliberal societies by which we assume that individuals make choices that guide their life biographies, including choices that make them "sick" or "healthy." Women, who are depicted in this discourse as fully autonomous and rational individuals, are morally responsible for being aware of the risk factors and for taking steps to reduce them. Women's responsibility for making choices—a moral responsibility—is delineated most clearly on the ACS web site. For each risk factor the ACS lists as a lifestyle choice, it offers a recommendation statement. For example, "The American Cancer Society suggests limiting the amount you drink to one drink a day."[37] In this model, women who are responsible and follow the guidelines for action regain control over their future, purportedly one free of breast cancer. Unfortunately, as Fosket notes, "identifying and eliminating a factor associated with increased cancer risk does not necessarily translate into disease prevention."[38] Even if women attempt to reduce or eliminate all lifestyle risk factors, they do not eliminate the possibility of breast cancer in their future. This framing of risks as controllable contributes to a certain neoliberal form of self-discipline. Managing risk becomes, as Komen for the Cure suggests, as much an everyday activity as wearing seat belts and brushing one's teeth.[39]

Unavoidable/unchangeable risks are often more clearly situated in the body, although the body is also implicated in the representation of lifestyle risks. Nikolas Rose suggests that "we are increasingly coming to relate to ourselves as 'somatic' individuals, that is to say, as beings whose individuality is, in part at least, grounded within our fleshly, corporeal existence, and who experience, articulate, judge, and act upon ourselves in part in the language of biomedicine."[40] As such, popular discourses of risk such as those the ACS, the NCI, and Komen for the Cure present take part in the "increasing stress on personal reconstruction through acting on the body in the name of a fitness that is simultaneously corporeal and psychological. . . . The corporeal existence and vitality of the self has become the privileged site of experiments with the self."[41] Given the focus on our selves as corporeal, it is not surprising that the urging of women to act in terms of managing risk also extends to clearly biological factors that are out of one's control. The ACS describes these factors, which include gender, age, race, family history, and genetics, as things "you cannot change."[42] The NCI frames similar issues as unavoidable: "For example, both smoking and inheriting certain genes are risk factors for some types of cancer, but only smoking can be avoided."[43] The focus of much of the discourse of uncontrollable risk is genetics—specifically the BRCA1 and BRCA2 gene mutations—although even Komen for the Cure admits that such mutations are rare (90 to 95 percent of breast cancer diagnoses do not involve a genetic mutation).[44]

Genetic risk is presented in a straightforward fashion on most mainstream web sites, although the statistics these sites offer vary. Komen for the Cure offers a lengthy explanation of the BRCA1 and BRCA2 mutations:

> Between 1 in 400 and 1 in 800 women in the U.S. are BRCA1 or BRCA2 carriers. Women who carry a BRCA1 or BRCA2 genetic mutation have a much higher risk of breast cancer. A woman's chance of getting breast

cancer in her lifetime (assuming she lives until the age of 85) is about 12 percent if she does not have a BRCA1/2 mutation. For women who carry a BRCA1 or BRCA2 gene mutation, estimates of breast cancer risk vary greatly. The lifetime risk of breast cancer for BRCA1 carriers ranges from 60 to 90 percent. For BRCA2 carriers, estimates range from 30 to 85 percent.[45]

The actions women take once they are situated as having a high lifetime risk of breast cancer is shaped by the discourse of prevention that circulates in survivor culture. The attention paid to genetics on the ACS, NCI, and Komen for the Cure web sites reflects a substantial shift in medicine since the advent of "personalized medicine" that is made possible through genomics and the study of hereditary factors in disease.[46] This shift has "consequences for the ways in which individuals are governed, and the ways in which they govern themselves."[47] As Rose explains, "The reorganization of many illnesses and pathologies along a genetic axis does not generate fatalism. On the contrary, it creates an obligation to act in the present in relation to the potential futures that now come into view."[48] Adding the science of genetics to the rhetoric of risk surrounding breast cancer does not change the overall message of choice and personal responsibility because as neoliberal subjects always engaged in the process of perfecting the self, genetically risky individuals are not reduced to passive body-machines. Instead, by making an unwanted future knowable, the discourses of genetic risk "seem to invite or even demand medical intervention on the susceptible individual in the present to direct his or her path to a different, and more desirable—less diseased—future."[49] Elisabeth Beck-Gernsheim offers one interpretation of the "demand for medical intervention," suggesting that new gene technology promotes an understanding of health that is based on individual genetic risk factors as guidelines for shaping lifestyles. These guidelines, she argues, quickly become "preventative compulsions" that guide patients' choices.[50]

Discourse from organizations about genetic risk and breast cancer—including the ACS, NCI, and Komen web sites—aligns with Beck-Gernsheim's assertions: testing positive for one of the BRCA gene mutations in this discourse positions women as "previvors" who are now enabled to make a compulsory choice regarding prevention. The term previvor was formulated by a group called FORCE (Facing Our Risk of Cancer Empowered), which defines such women as "individuals who are sur*vivors* of a *pre*disposition to *cancer* but who haven't had the disease."[51] The previvor identity is based fundamentally on an optimistic view of life and science and the belief that once an individual is empowered to make choices, cancer can be conquered or simply avoided altogether. Not acting—or not attempting to manage one's risk—is not one of the options open to previvors. Previvors are offered three specific options for prevention. The first—heightened surveillance—offers women the choice of undergoing mammograms and MRI scans on a frequent schedule (as often as every six months). Popular press accounts of the surveillance option suggests that this option is not attractive as it does very little to ease women's fear of getting cancer and also involves a constant heightened awareness of the potential of having cancer. A *New York Times* article on the rise in prophylactic double mastectomies offers this explanation from Dr. Todd Tuttle, a surgical oncologist: "The comment patients make is, 'I just want to be done with it.' . . . They never want to have another mammogram again; they never want to have another biopsy again."[52]

A second avenue for previvors is chemoprevention, which broadly refers to the use of medication to lower one's risk. Tamoxifen is the most widely used drug for chemoprevention, and the ACS and Komen for the Cure web sites offer discussions of both the risks and benefits of Tamoxifen. However, the ACS supports the use of Tamoxifen: "The drug Tamoxifen has already been used for many years as a treatment for some types of breast cancer. Studies have shown that women at high risk for breast cancer are less likely to get the disease if they take tamoxifen."[53] This simple statement omits the fact that chemoprevention is still a highly controversial practice; some European studies have found no reduction in the incidence of breast cancer among women taking Tamoxifen.[54] Fosket expands on the problem: "Within the United States, these discrepancies [between U.S. and European studies] are commonly explained away as the result of too few numbers in the European studies, confounding factors . . . , differential compliance, and different conceptualizations of 'high risk.' . . . In contrast, many European reports depict the North American Breast Cancer Prevention Trial, especially its early unmasking and publication of results on the internet, as prematurely optimistic, or, worse, as bad science."[55] Framed by the repeated statistics and objective tone of both the ACS and Komen web sites, the informed decision to pursue chemoprevention is discussed as the "right choice" for some women at high risk.[56] Remarkably, Jennifer Fosket suggests that one of the reasons for chemoprevention's reputation as a reasonable solution for high-risk women is the nonviability of prophylactic surgery as a widespread prevention method.[57] She explains that "removing one's breasts for the potential prevention of a potential disease carries with it physical, social, and psychological risks of numerous kinds, and thus the procedure remains quite controversial."[58]

Despite these problems, prophylactic mastectomies, the third option for previvors, have been the subject of increasing news coverage. The assertion that "bilateral prophylactic mastectomy will almost always prevent the development of breast cancer" has proven to be persuasive with many women.[59] One *New York Times* headline declares "Study Finds Rise in Choice of Double Mastectomies," and a ABC News headline echoed the message, "More Women Choosing 'Preventive' Double Mastectomy."[60] Prophylactic mastectomies are represented as the most effective way of reducing risk for BRCA1 and BRCA2 carriers because the procedure reduces breast cancer risk by approximately 90 to 95 percent.[61] Both Komen and the ACS caution women not to move forward too quickly with surgery (Komen reminds its readers that there "is no need to rush"), but as the Komen web site notes, "[The surgery] may also make women feel that they have done all they can do to prevent [cancer]. Studies suggest that prophylactic bilateral mastectomy can lower the risk of breast cancer in women at high risk by 90 percent or more."[62] When genetic breast cancer risk is framed as actionable, the compulsion to act, to change the future for the better, is clear. Young women, Komen reports, may see the greatest benefits from surgery as they "have more years of life ahead of them than older women."[63] It is precisely those years (often years that are active in terms of both reproduction and sexuality) that women who have tested positive for the BRCA1 and BRCA2 mutations are encouraged to claim for themselves. Prophylactic mastectomies seem to hold for women the promise of a cancer-free future. The construction of prophylactic mastectomy as a "compulsory choice" in public discourse relies both on the framing of genetic risks as "actionable" and the careful construction of a particular subject—the cancer/risk-free woman—to which I turn next.

Embodied Risk and the Empowered Postfeminist Subject

Two of the most visible public stories of prophylactic mastectomies are those of Christina Applegate and Jessica Queller. As examples of mainstream public discourse, the texts of the Queller and Applegate narratives are strikingly similar, although there is one difference. Queller's narrative focuses on her bilateral prophylactic mastectomy, a procedure in which a cancer-free woman has both breasts removed. Applegate's narrative details her experience with a contralateral prophylactic mastectomy, or the removal of both breasts in the case where breast cancer is present in only one breast. The rate of contralateral prophylactic mastectomies has risen significantly in recent years, from 1.8 percent in 1998 to 4.8 percent in 2003, in part because of statistics suggesting that women who have cancer in one breast have a 2 to 11 percent chance of cancer occurring in their second breast.[64] Bilateral prophylactic mastectomies are more rare but are nevertheless an important subject of interest for both the public and for women who test positive for a BRCA gene mutation. For example, in one study comparing rates of contralateral and bilateral prophylactic mastectomies, of the 128 patients who had prophylactic mastectomies in a two-year period at Saint Barnabas Medical Center in New Jersey, 103 patients had a contralateral prophylactic mastectomy, compared to 21 patients who had a bilateral prophylactic mastectomy (4 patients were excluded).[65] Marlene Frost notes that 16 to 20 percent of women at high risk for breast cancer rate prophylactic bilateral mastectomy as a favorable option, and Meijers-Heijboer and colleagues report a "high demand" for both genetic testing and prophylactic surgeries in a clinical setting.[66] The difference between contralateral and bilateral prophylactic mastectomies disappears in the narratives of Jessica Queller and Christina Applegate; they are both reported and discussed through a discourse of risk that equates having the BRCA1 or BRCA2 gene mutation with having cancer.

Jessica Queller is a television writer for shows such as *Gossip Girl* and *Gilmore Girls*, and her memoir describing her bilateral prophylactic mastectomy was a best seller. My analysis of Queller's narrative uses her memoir as a primary text but also includes the commentary offered in book reviews and the numerous interviews Queller gave on the publicity circuit for her memoir. The narrative about Applegate's contralateral prophylactic mastectomy is constructed by the entertainment press. The discourse I analyze comes from numerous sources, including the entertainment coverage of Applegate and her interviews with Robin Roberts on *Good Morning America* and with Oprah Winfrey. In addition, I draw from a variety of news and popular media stories to supplement the voices of Queller and Applegate, including news profiles of other women who have had bilateral prophylactic mastectomies. My analysis of the prophylactic mastectomy narrative—using Applegate and Queller as touchstones—suggests that women who test positive for a BRCA gene mutation are represented as empowered health citizens who can claim their bodies, rid their bodies of risk, and reconstruct their bodies to fit a new, cancer/risk-free subjectivity. I begin by discussing the role of cancer risk in the prophylactic mastectomy narrative, arguing that any risk related breast cancer is represented as unacceptable. I then move to a discussion of the ways the identity of the cancer/risk-free woman combines a postfeminist discourse of empowerment and choice with a biomedicalization of risk that creates two distinct realms of breast cancer patients—those who have been empowered and are no longer vulnerable (they are risk free), and those who are disempowered and at risk—that break down along class and race lines. Although I am critical of the implications of this narrative, I should reiterate that my criticism is reserved for the narrative—that is, the ways women and their choices are represented in public discourse—and is not aimed at the decisions that women such as Applegate and Queller make when facing a positive result from a genetic test.

Framing Cancer as an Unacceptable Risk

A lengthy *New York Times* article published in September 2007 described the agonizing decision made by Deborah Linder, then thirty-three, to have a bilateral prophylactic mastectomy after testing positive for the BRCA1 mutation.[67] As a single, healthy woman who was finishing medical school, Linder was concerned about a variety of issues related to having a prophylactic mastectomy: the ability to find a partner after having her breasts removed, her inability to ever breastfeed if she chose to have children, and the potential complications of the surgery. However, her biggest fear lay in the specter of cancer. Ms. Linder was already enrolled in an intensive surveillance program, and she recalls that her vulnerability to cancer literally took over her mind; she was spending her days worrying about breast cancer, examining her breasts, and researching statistics and possible options. In addition to cancer—which for women in the Linder family had resulted in numerous deaths and prolonged battles—the article suggests that treatments were also a source of Ms. Linder's anxiety: "Deborah remembered her mother's cancer diagnosis, which came just before her graduation from high school. . . . During that summer, her mother's bedroom door, always open, stayed closed."[68] Ms. Linder notes that the effects of chemotherapy aged her mother in many subtle ways. Thus, she declares, "I don't want that for myself . . . I don't want to treat cancer. I just never want to get it."[69] Although this article is a single example of discourse about prophylactic mastectomies, it crafts a narrative—one of fear, determination, and the promise of liberation from cancer—that is mirrored in the narratives of Applegate and Queller. Within the prophylactic mastectomy narrative, the line between genetic risk and cancer is blurred and the experience of having cancer (not simply being diagnosed with cancer) is emphasized. Faced with what becomes an unacceptable risk, both Queller and Applegate are represented as empowered citizens who stake their claim to being women who are free of both cancer and the risk of cancer.

Genes and Cancer

In the iteration of the vulnerable empowered woman presented in the prophylactic mastectomy narrative, each woman's vulnerability is configured as her embodied risk (her genetic risk) for cancer. The line between testing positive for the BRCA1 and BRCA2 gene mutation and being diagnosed with cancer is consistently blurred in both the Queller and Applegate narratives, although the test result is not explicitly equated with having cancer. Queller's memoir, *Pretty Is What Changes: Impossible Choices, the Breast Cancer Gene, and How I Defied My Destiny*, begins with a phone conversation with her doctor in which he announces her positive test result and explains that "statistically, you have up to an eighty-five or ninety percent chance of getting breast cancer."[70] Queller's memoir traces her decision to have a prophylactic double mastectomy through a structure that ignores linear chronology. After an introduction in which Queller tests positive for the BRCA mutation in 2004, the first chapter moves back in time to 2001 where Queller finds herself sitting in a hospital with her mother and sister, watching as her grandmother slowly succumbs to kidney failure. A few months later, complaining of stomach pain, her mother visits the hospital and is diagnosed with stage IIIC ovarian cancer and is given a prognosis of five years to live. Queller relates that six years earlier, her mother had been diagnosed with and then "beaten" breast cancer. Much of Queller's memoir focuses on her mother's journey with cancer and cancer treatments, a point to which I return below. What is key in terms of the blurring of "having a gene" and "having cancer" is the overall structure of Queller's narrative. That is, by beginning the memoir with a positive test result but then immediately moving to the past to reflect on her mother's experience with cancer, the positive test is associated closely—both textually and emotionally—with having cancer.

After her mother's death, Queller decides to take the genetic test but does not think seriously about the possible consequences. She remembers that instead of talking with genetic counselors before taking the test, she opted to take the test at a lab where no questions were asked, explaining, "I was so convinced I would test negative that I didn't feel I had to bother with any of those steps."[71] Later, with her positive results finally in hand, Queller gives the specific statistics: "Deleterious mutations in BRCA1 may confer as much as an 87 percent risk of breast cancer and a 44 percent risk of ovarian cancer by the age of 70 in women."[72] Queller's narrative frames the meaning of the risk with her personal experience of her mother's cancer. She remembers, "In spite of the fact that my mother had cancer twice, I did not feel the disease would ever strike *me*. I had witnessed the horror of cancer up close. I knew my mother had been shocked each time she'd been seized by cancer. And yet, strangely, I felt invincible."[73] However, once she tested positive for the BRCA1 gene, Queller's views change. She is no longer invincible; she is vulnerable. Queller feels an "ominous chill" that is the result of the statistics that suggest she is at a high lifetime risk of getting breast cancer and the implicit message of medical personnel, genetic counselors, and her own history with her mother: if you don't have cancer now, you will.[74] In this formulation, there is no "85 percent chance" of having cancer; instead, the chance is 100 percent, a certainty that once one has the mutation, one will have cancer.

The formulation of cancer as "destiny" (taking a cue from the title of her book) and unavoidable once one tests positive for the BRCA mutation is seen in Queller's surroundings when she visits her genetic counselor. She stands in line to sign in at the reception desk behind a bald woman in a scarf. In the parking garage, she sees another woman with a bald head. Signs of cancer surround Queller, and having been tested, she is clearly situated as a member of the cancer regime. Maren Klawiter notes that one of the results of the transformation of breast cancer culture into one that emphasizes routine screening and early detection is the increase in the numbers of women participating in the "breast cancer continuum." Women with normal mammograms, women with abnormal mammograms, women with biopsies, women with false positives, women with ductal carcinoma in situ, women with cancer are all constituted as vulnerable and at-risk subjects.[75] The discovery of the BRCA1 and BRCA2 genes and the increase in genetic testing has increased the number of cancer-free women participating in breast cancer culture as at-risk subjects. However, in Queller's story, she is not merely an at-risk subject; she is always already a woman with cancer. On the day of her genetic counseling, Queller has a sonogram that finds a breast cyst. After close inspection by a doctor, the cyst is determined to be benign, but it nevertheless raises the specter of cancer. Her friend Kay reinforces the conflation of a positive test with cancer, explaining that her own breast surgeon treats women with the BRCA1 gene mutation as breast cancer patients.[76] Journalist Masha Gessen experienced a similar phenomenon after her positive test result for the BRCA1 mutation. Gessen remembers that like the patients of Kay's breast surgeon, she became a "professional patient," one who would also be ill until proven healthy.[77]

Perhaps the clearest way that having the breast cancer gene is equated with having cancer is through a series of anecdotes Queller offers in which women who test positive for the BRCA1 or BRCA2 mutation already have cancer, although they may not know it, or women who are diagnosed with breast cancer turn out to be BRCA1 or BRCA2 carriers. Consider, for example, Queller's telling of the story of Kerry, a woman who discovered a lump in her breast at the age of thirty-four. Kerry has a mastectomy and decides on her own to have the BRCA test, although her doctors discourage it. Queller describes the results: "Her instincts were right—she tested positive for BRCA-1. Soon after, a spot was found on her ovaries."[78] Queller also relates the story of Sue Friedman, the eventual founder of FORCE, who was diagnosed with breast cancer at the age of 33 and then, after reading about the BRCA mutations, was tested and received a positive test result.[79] Even before testing positive for the BRCA mutation, both Kerry and Friedman are already breast cancer patients. They are never only BRCA positive. Queller's own story confirms the conflation of the gene with cancer. She relates, "Two weeks after the surgery, I went in to see Dr. Roses for an exam. He held the pathology report in his hand. 'You had precancerous changes in your right breast tissue, Jessica. Atypical ductal hyperplasia.' I was shocked. 'If you had any doubt about the course of action you chose, this should dispel it. You did the right thing.'"[80] The doctor's remarks are worth a close look. First, running throughout the narratives is a postfeminist discourse of choice and the empowerment that comes from choice. Here, we see a doctor applauding Queller for making the "right choice." Second, I would suggest that the doctor's findings confirm for Queller—and the public—that the embodied risk of the BRCA gene for getting cancer is not a risk at all—it is a certainty. Queller's surgery (officially a bilateral prophylactic mastectomy) is transformed with her new "pre-cancer" diagnosis into a procedure that resembles a contralateral prophylactic mastectomy, or the removal of both breasts when cancer has been found in only one.

The blurring of the gene and cancer occurs in a slightly different formula in the Applegate narrative, but the certainty about cancer is the same. What is significant for Applegate's story is the time line offered to the public through press releases and interviews Applegate gave. Applegate announced her cancer diagnosis in early August 2008. Her publicist explained, "Benefitting from early detection through a doctor-ordered MRI, the cancer is not life threatening."[81] Reuters reported that Applegate was "following the recommended treatment of her doctors" and would have a full recovery.[82] Over the next two weeks, the Applegate story faded from public view, although there was some speculation about what type of treatment Applegate was having. A new dimension of the story broke with Applegate's August 19 interview with Robin Roberts on ABC. In this interview, Applegate explained that her original treatment regimen—two lumpectomies and radiation—had been altered significantly. She had undergone a "double prophylactic mastectomy" because she had tested positive for the BRCA gene.[83] Applegate explained to Oprah later in September that "I tested positive for the BRCA gene and that changed everything for me, because radiation was really just something temporary that wasn't addressing the issue of this coming back."[84] What is significant about the Applegate narrative is that her cancer diagnosis occurred before she received the positive test results for the BRCA gene mutation. With the public confirmation of her BRCA status, Applegate enacted the disappearing line between having the gene mutation and having cancer—by the time she discovered her BRCA status, she was already a cancer patient. Like the anecdotes Queller shared, and indeed like Queller herself, Applegate never had the opportunity to be simply "BRCA positive."

Emphasizing the Cancer Experience

The second way that cancer is formulated as an unacceptable risk is through the emphasis on the cancer experience: the treatments, the side effects, and the uncertainty. This often occurs as a result of remembering the cancer experiences of close relatives—mothers, sisters, aunts, daughters. The experience of cancer is often undeniably traumatic; while treatments may extend life, they come with varying noxious side effects. Trauma specialists suggest that breast cancer may be a particularly traumatic illness: "Breast cancer may have somewhat unique psychological effects compared to other cancer diagnoses. It is disproportionately a health problem of women; its treatment and course is often uncertain; and its treatment can include visible disfigurement. Given the chronic nature of being diagnosed with, treated for, and living with cancer, it may entail both a threat to life and an ongoing threat to quality of life."[85] Gessen reflects on one young woman's insistence on having both a preventive double mastectomy and an oophorectomy: "She had seen her mother live through a debilitating course of treatment at the age of thirty-four and again at forty-two. What drove her was not even so much a fear of death as a fear of cancer as a way of life—her family's way of life."[86] The desire to avoid the experience of cancer is clear in the narratives of both Queller and Applegate.

Applegate remembers watching her mother, a "quiet warrior," go through "two years of chemotherapy and eight surgeries and a hysterectomy."[87] Robin Roberts, the ABC interviewer, describes Applegate's mother, Nancy Priddy, in celebratory tones, noting, for example, that Applegate had witnessed Priddy "handle it [breast cancer] beautifully" and that Priddy has been a "special source of strength" for Applegate during her difficult time.[88] Applegate echoes

Roberts's admiration of her mother, suggesting that after watching her mother survive years of chemotherapy and multiple surgeries, she always knew that "I was gonna be okay no matter what."[89] These celebratory memories, however, are somewhat dampened by what Roberts calls Applegate's "most important real-life role": caring for her mother with cancer—not once, but twice. Roberts explains that this was "a role that made her vigilant about screening for the disease, a vigilance that helped doctors catch her breast cancer early and led to Christina's dramatic choice of treatment."[90] Applegate's personal experience with prolonged cancer treatment is a key factor behind her decision to have the prophylactic mastectomy: "I just wanted to kind of be rid of this whole thing for me."[91]

Much of Queller's memoir is devoted to describing her mother's experiences with cancer in grim detail. Queller's mother's death is traumatic—her long battle with cancer is an experience that leaves both Queller and her sister Danielle "shaking from trauma."[92] Queller explains her choice to go forward with her prophylactic mastectomy to Cokie Roberts: "I spoke to many oncologists around the country, one of whom was your doctor, and I think it was she who told me it really is a personal choice; it's a question of your tolerance for fighting breast cancer. . . . My answer is that having watched my mother die a brutal, horrific death—to me, cancer is the worst thing in the world, I don't want to gamble with it."[93] In the prophylactic mastectomy narrative, an undeniable part of what makes the experience of cancer so traumatic for both patients and their families is how the American medical industry treats cancer. Queller's mother's death follows a painful, horrifying year of chemotherapy, surgeries, radiation, drug cocktails, and the multitude of side effects that result from modern cancer treatments. Queller narrates her mother's heartbreaking final days: "The following day, September 20, 2003, my mother's lungs filled with fluid. Every breath she took was like drowning. The thick, heavy, gurgling sound of her gasping breaths will forever haunt me. My mother's eyes were filled with terror, her mouth frozen in a permanent O. She refused to get near the bed—and insisted on walking. . . . My father looked on, helpless and aghast. 'She doesn't deserve this,' he said. 'My bride was stunning. So beautiful.' The last words of my mother's I could understand were 'Help,' and 'This is against my will.'"[94] The focus on the experience of cancer continues in the words of one FORCE member in a letter written to Queller: "Cancer of any kind should not be considered an option, but a horrific, life-changing event, occurring without our consent. I'm currently in treatment and have watched my mom and five of her siblings suffer through their treatments, some successfully, some not.

Bravo to you, Jessica, for choosing NOT to take the risk/option of cancer."[95] In this discourse, the side effects of treatment are literally effects of cancer. The emphasis on the experience of cancer—the experience of both the cancer patient and those of her caretakers—serves to enhance the fear and dread felt by women with BRCA mutations. This emotional state, along with the collapsing of the BRCA gene mutation into having cancer, is key in the construction of the method of empowerment for the cancer/risk-free woman in which cancer is no longer an option.

The Cancer/Risk-Free Woman

Both the collapsing of the BRCA gene into having cancer and the emphasis on the experience of cancer narrated through memories of loved ones situate cancer as an unacceptable risk and propel certain actions. That is, the absolute destiny of cancer for women with the BRCA gene mutation and the inevitable pain, misery, and grief brought on by cancer as presented in this discourse necessitate empowerment through the "dramatic," "brave" and "radical" decision to have a prophylactic double mastectomy.[96] Both the Queller and Applegate narratives articulate a justification in which actions such as prophylactic mastectomies are framed as "logical" (to use Applegate's description) based on the need to avoid future incidences of breast cancer at all costs. Indeed, avoiding future cancer becomes the singular focus of the cancer/risk-free woman, and while I am critical of compulsory "choice" that in this narrative is the result of the desire to avoid cancer, such avoidance is all too understandable given the trauma of cancer and cancer treatment. Expressions of this characteristic can be found in both Applegate's and Queller's stories. Applegate explains, "I didn't want to go back to the doctors every four months for testing and squishing and everything"[97] and "I don't want next year to have to deal with this again."[98] Applegate reflects on her post-mastectomy, cancer-free body: "I'm clear, absolutely 100 percent clear and clean. It did not spread. They got everything out. So I'm definitely not gonna die from breast cancer. . . . Maybe a bus but, you know, I really—that I have nothing to do with."[99] Applegate's description of her lack of breast cancer risk contradicts medical reports that suggest that while prophylactic mastectomies reduce one's cancer risk (by up to 98 percent), they do not eliminate all risk because it is difficult to remove all breast tissue. In addition, through her comparison of the risk of breast cancer with the risk of being hit by a bus, her description confirms that certain behaviors are expected when individuals are faced with a genetic risk. While Applegate cannot limit her risk of being hit by a bus, her BRCA status compelled her to make a decision to avoid the risk of cancer at any cost so she could have a healthy future.

Similarly, Queller feels that until people understand her story—in particular her experiences with her mother—they cannot fully appreciate the choice she made. In an interview with *US News*, Queller explains that after she tested positive for the BRCA gene mutation, she "was in denial about how serious my situation was" until she did her own research and "learned about BRCA-positive women getting cancer in their 30s."[100] Her reasoning echoes that of Applegate's appeal to logic and rationality. Her research suggested that she had two possible courses of action: vigilant screening or mastectomy. Queller explains to Cokie Roberts her decision to have a double mastectomy: "I don't want to gamble that maybe we'll catch it early enough. After going through a long, long process I came to the decision that I would do anything I needed to prevent it in the first place."[101] Queller opts to rid herself of the risk. As she writes in her memoir, "Was there a point in doing surveillance, waiting for cancer to strike, and then getting a mastectomy anyway? In that case, I would have to live with the threat of recurrence—that one renegade cancer cell had been left behind and would resurface somewhere else in my body. Was that worth a few more years of natural breasts?"[102] Near the end of her book, Queller declares triumphantly, but in somber tone: "I am now thirty-seven, with the perilous threat of breast cancer behind me and the threat of ovarian cancer still looming. I will have my ovaries prophylactically removed at forty."[103] In an extensive *Los Angeles Times* article, Queller evokes what is so central to the identity of the cancer/risk-free woman: the freedom from cancer. "Everything is tenable except for illness. If I lose my job, if I get my heart broken, if—God forbid—I can't have a child, I will be devastated, but whatever it is, I can deal with it. Anything but illness is OK."[104]

The Politics of Choice: Risk-Free or Risky Living?

The stories of Queller and Applegate revolve around the theme of choice and variations on that theme: empowerment, taking action, and taking control. Perhaps appropriately, the *New York Times* story on Deborah Linder's choice received numerous letters to the editor, including Susan K. Cashen's letter: "I'm a BRCA1 carrier and like Deborah Linder, the subject of your article, I addressed my risk by opting for surgery. It was an easy decision, one that was supported by my husband, family and friends. Having watched my mother battle ovarian cancer, I wanted to fight the cancer beast on my own terms, proactively. I didn't want to struggle for my life, afraid and weakened not only by a hideous disease, but by the treatment necessary to kill it."[105] The emphasis on knowledge, taking action, being proactive, and choosing what is best for you and your body all reflect the central themes of empowerment and bodily self-determination that guided the women's health movement. These themes are ubiquitous in discussions of women's health today. However, although these messages sound much the same as they did in the 1970s, when they are placed in a neoliberal, postfeminist context, the message of empowerment has substantially different implications. Women's empowerment in the prophylactic mastectomy narrative depends on their ability and willingness to fully engage in biomedical culture and consume medical services as the primary way to ensure a healthy future. The postfeminist logic of the prophylactic mastectomy narrative emerges most clearly through two elements of prophylactic mastectomy narratives: first, they situate the choice to have mastectomies within a moralized discourse of risk; and second, they envision an idealized white, female body that can be (re)constructed through surgery.

Prophylactic Mastectomies and Moralized Risk

In her memoir and related interviews, Queller repeatedly insists that the decision to have a prophylactic double mastectomy is a highly personal one. She explains to *Newsweek*, "But it's very important to me not to proselytize. . . . There are tons of young people who have the gene but say they're just not ready to make the decision."[106] Despite such explicit statements, the choice to have a prophylactic mastectomy is firmly situated within a highly moralized construction of risk. In the prophylactic mastectomy narrative, a clear "right choice" and "wrong choice" emerge. Rhetorics of risk are almost always grounded in moral issues, in part because risk "is primarily understood as a human responsibility, both in its production and management, rather than the outcome of fate or destiny."[107] The moral foundations of risk discourse are particularly apparent in relation to health, where choices made in relation to risk factors invite a sense of "human mastery over disease" that, when exercised properly, can result in the avoidance of any/all illness.[108]

Information about breast cancer is thoroughly saturated with discourses of personal responsibility, including information regarding the embodied risk of BRCA gene mutations. The narrative about prophylactic mastectomies continues in this trend, for despite the explicit references to the importance of each woman making her own choice in the narrative, the rightness or wrongness of each choice is made apparent through the anecdotes and asides. Consider the format of *Newsweek*'s recommendations: "Ultimately, of course, it's an incredibly personal choice, one that women should make carefully, evaluating all the information available. Rachel Meiser's aunt, Chari Briggs-Krenis, sixty-nine, who also has the CDH1 genetic mutation, had her breasts removed twenty-six years ago. 'I read these things about people whose whole life seems to hang on having breasts,' she says. 'These are attachments that one can easily live without.' She, like many who've taken the difficult road of double mastectomy, says she has no second thoughts."[109] Although *Newsweek* begins with a routine statement that "it's a personal choice," the final sentence of the article offers a judgment by quoting a woman who has "no second thoughts" about her own prophylactic mastectomy. She made the right choice. Similarly, in a letter to the editor of *USA Today*, a woman named Nirenejca explains the many reasons why keeping her breasts, what she describes as "healthy ticking time bombs," was not an option and declares, "I chose to be proactive because I'm not a dumb gambler."[110] Both Briggs-Krenis and Nirenejca suggest that women's focus on keeping breasts is misguided. The many references to women who have had positive experiences with prophylactic mastectomies colors the choices available to women with BRCA gene mutations. It is notable, for example, that in my extensive review of the public discourse about prophylactic mastectomies, I could not find a single example of a woman expressing regret about her decision to remove her breasts.

Postfeminist constructions of women's agency are an important part of the moral overtones associated with women's choices to have a prophylactic mastectomy. As represented in the prophylactic mastectomy narrative, a woman's choice is informed by both discourses of individuality and traditional womanhood. Both Applegate and Queller's stories echo the rhetoric of the women's health movement: their health is important because they are important; their own well-being is reason enough for staying healthy. Queller and Applegate repeatedly make statements about their desires not to repeat their mothers' experiences, and these statements can be interpreted as a declaration of individual health and well-being. Nevertheless, it is difficult for their narratives to escape discussion of traditional expectations for women, specifically regarding motherhood and marriage. In a voice-over during her interview with Applegate, Robin Roberts explains Applegate's reasons for the interview: "She wasn't really ready to go public yet, but there was some false reporting . . . saying that she was putting off chemotherapy to start a family, that she really wanted to get pregnant. She does want to have a family one day, but that is not the reason she made her choice."[111] Family issues are a frequent part of the prophylactic mastectomy narrative, in part because many of the women facing the decision are young, single, and childless. As Gessen notes, "For modern women, particularly western Jewish professional ones who have children later, the mutation may bring cancer before the child-rearing years are past."[112] Queller deals with the issue of reproduction extensively in her memoir, sharing her concerns that having a prophylactic double mastectomy would decrease her ability to find a life partner. But, like Applegate, she explicitly rejects the issue of "family" as a reason for having or not having a prophylactic mastectomy. In her interview with Cokie Roberts, Queller recalls her discomfort at the focus on her personal life, including this comment by Cokie Roberts: "Talk about pressure! I mean the biological clock ticks, but it's ticking very loud."[113] Queller's response is telling: "Yes, that is very upsetting and distressing to me. . . . But I've come to peace with the mastectomy and I'm also at peace with the idea of having a child or two in the next five years, and if I have to do it on my own, I will do it on my own."[114] The representation of Queller's position is in many ways a perfect condensation of the postfeminist position on reproduction. Tasker and Negra explain, "Women's lives are regularly conceived of as time starved; women themselves are overworked, rushed, harassed, subject to their 'biological clocks,' and so on to such a degree that female adulthood is defined as a state of chronic temporal crisis."[115] Queller's calm façade in response to a reminder that she is dealing with a "ticking clock" is undermined by her sense of urgency about starting a family.

Although the Applegate and Queller narratives support women making the right choice for themselves—with the promise of a happy heterosexual family life in the future—other women's voices in public discourse about prophylactic mastectomies complicate this position. What emerges is a dual logic that crafts one line of reasoning for childless women and another line of reasoning for women with children. In Queller's memoir, the "woman with child" figure is represented by her sister, Danielle. Although Danielle expresses horror in the beginning of the memoir at Queller's decision to have a bilateral prophylactic mastectomy, Danielle's position softens when she too tests positive for the BRCA gene mutation. Unlike Jessica, Danielle is happily married and has a newborn when she discovers her BRCA status. Queller explains her sister's new position: "Now that she had a baby, Dani felt an enormous responsibility to remain healthy. She would have the mastectomy."[116] Queller also tells the story of a friend who decided to take the BRCA test: "Alexandra had a baby boy, Sam, shortly after Danielle had Miles. Once she had a child, she, too, felt the pressure to protect her health. Alex had been a young girl when she witnessed her mother die of cancer—she did not want her son to endure the same horror."[117] Both Danielle and Alexandra (who tested negative for the BRCA mutation) made decisions that were influenced by feelings of responsibility for and pressure to take care of others.

As Queller and Applegate are represented as standing up for their own health, the supporting characters in their stories are represented as taking a stand for others, expressing the need to be there for their children and their larger families. Although the motivations may seem different, I suggest that they are actually quite similar: the choice of treatment is made in order to make possible or protect an already existing relationship with a child. Queller's focus on finding the "right man" (readers are introduced to three boyfriends in her memoir) and having children, including her decision to use in vitro fertilization at the end of the book when she is still not in a long-term relationship, point to a key reason for her decision to have a prophylactic mastectomy: her desire to have a family. She explains her focus on her "ticking clock" to Sarah Bernard of *New York Magazine*: "I didn't have the luxury of being someone in her early thirties dating and falling in love and being free."[118] Instead, doctors advised removing her ovaries when she was forty, offering her a few years to become pregnant with or without a life partner. Queller argues at the end of her book that "we are living in an age in which scientific advances give us new opportunities to live. Seize them."[119] Yet the choice Queller is empowered to make places her in a double bind. On the one hand, having a prophylactic double mastectomy (followed in a few years by the removal of her ovaries) may make her goal of finding a life partner and having children more difficult. She explains her original response to her doctor's advice to Renée Montagne in an interview on National Public Radio: "I'm single and dating and I want a family, and I would never consider—I mean, it was an outrageous proposition to me at the time. . . . I had terrible fears that I would feel deformed . . . that I wouldn't be attractive to men as a single woman."[120] On the other hand, without the surgery—given the formulation that equates the BRCA gene mutation with an inevitable cancer diagnosis—the family Queller desires would not be possible at all.

The characterization of choice in the prophylactic mastectomy narrative is a unique combination of a rhetoric of risk that gives all individuals the power (and the responsibility) to make choices in their lives and a postfeminist context in which those choices are crafted to appeal to women's sense of empowerment and yet continue to reify one of the most traditional aspects of being a woman: motherhood. In a review of Queller's memoir for the *Los Angeles Times*, Diana Wagman suggests that Queller had "too many choices" to make—to have the genetic test or not, to tell friends and family or not, to have surgery or not, to opt for surveillance or not—choices which are not available to women after they have had cancer.[121] However, I would suggest that Queller's narrative, and that of Applegate, Deborah Linder, and the many other women who are featured in mainstream public discourse, empower women to make only one choice. In the end, it is a choice that offers a promise of a cancer/risk-free identity and a fulfilling family life, complete with children and husband.

Transforming Body and Identity

The identity of the cancer/risk-free woman crafted through the prophylactic mastectomy narrative is based upon not simply making the right choice in the face of an unacceptable risk but on the false assumption that all women can make that choice. The emphasis on choice ignores the reality that many women with breast cancer do not have choice. As of 2007, over seventeen million women in the United States did not have health insurance.[122] That the choice made by Queller and Applegate to have prophylactic mastectomies is naturalized and universalized points to one of the key characteristics of postfeminist culture: the focus on the experience of white, upper-middle-class women. Tasker and Negra argue that postfeminism "participates in the ideological and economic normalization of new patterns of exclusion and demographic propriety in the United States and the United Kingdom."[123] The focus on elite women is clear in the detailed descriptions of the numerous surgeries, tests, and doctor's visits undertaken by women with the BRCA gene mutation as they craft a risk-free identity.

Both Applegate and Queller are privileged to the extent that they could afford genetic tests, frequent mammograms and MRIs, prophylactic surgery (which is not covered by all insurance programs), and extensive reconstructive surgery (which is rarely covered by insurance). Both are also privileged in terms of both race and class, as is evidenced by Applegate's presence as a television and movie actress and Queller's frequent references to her best friend Calista Flockhart (a well-known movie and television actress), her mother's house in the Hamptons, and her large collection of Manolo Blahnik shoes. Both also constitute the face of breast cancer that many scholars suggest is misleading: they are young (under forty), white, and wealthy. Even when the narrative explicitly recognizes health disparities (which are often based on class differences), it focuses on the women who already have the ability to make the right choice. The narrative paints a public image of women with BRCA gene mutations and/or family histories of breast cancer as young, white, and wealthy (and, for that matter, heterosexual) and assumes that all women can make the same choices.

Given the privileged and youthful status of the women who are articulated as cancer/risk-free women, it should come as no surprise that the prophylactic mastectomy narrative also features an unrelenting focus on appearance. Postfeminist culture celebrates disciplinary techniques focused on appearance such as cosmetic surgery, dieting, and wardrobe makeovers that encourage women to maintain a youthful femininity in terms of both physical appearance and attitude. The centrality of this postfeminist transformable body in prophylactic mastectomy discourse cannot be overstated. The postfeminist body reflects a dual understanding of women's bodies: "The body is presented simultaneously as women's source of power and as always unruly, requiring constant monitoring, surveillance, discipline, and remodeling (and consumer spending) in order to conform to ever-narrower judgments of female attractiveness."[124] In the prophylactic mastectomy narrative, two themes emerge in relation to transforming women's bodies that point to the specifically postfeminist logic at work: the promise of "good boobs" through new technology and the promise of a "better self" with better breasts. These themes center on the issue of beauty and reify the central place of breasts in defining femininity.

In a tone of relief, Christina Applegate remembers when she figured out that "they can make some pretty boobies, very pretty boobies."[125] Applegate's relief came hand in hand with her memory of her mother's mastectomy scar: "But that was back in the 70's and they didn't do it very good back then. . . . In my own mind I'm thinking, like, Oh my God, I'm going to be butchered and it's going to be horrible that I'm never gonna love my, you know, that part of me again."[126] Queller echoes her in a *US News* interview: "Plastic surgery is so advanced these days; they put you back together so beautifully. The brutal mastectomies of our mothers and grandmothers are simply not the case anymore."[127] Queller and Applegate construct a comparison of past and present that emphasizes new surgical methods and the need for women to love their breasts.

As Queller recounts, both the original mastectomy and the subsequent reconstructive surgeries (Queller had three surgeries in all) came with many options—how much skin and tissue to remove, whether or not to spare the nipples, what type of implants to choose, and so forth.[128] Questions about the future were important for both Queller and Applegate: "If I had a mastectomy and reconstruction, would men no longer find me desirable? Would I feel deformed? Would I ever want to be touched again? Would I no longer feel like a whole woman?"[129] These questions were answered through reference to the success of new surgical practices and the desirability of the results. Queller meets one young woman, a 35-year-old with two daughters, who had a double prophylactic mastectomy and hysterectomy because of her BRCA mutation: "Suzy took off her shirt. Her breasts looked astonishingly real. Of course, she had mastectomy scars, but they were faint. . . . Overall I felt heartened. Suzy didn't look scary or deformed—her breasts were beautiful. 'Touch them— don't they feel real?' We giggled as I touched my new friend's new fake boobs. 'Wow, they do feel real!' I said."[130] For Queller, Suzy's breasts hold the promise of retaining her attractiveness, and her concerns about her desirability post-mastectomy are diminished. These feelings are confirmed by her first long-term relationship after her surgery: "He often said he did not mourn the loss of my natural (and large) breasts—he loved the modest size I chose. He was a man who'd always been with gorgeous women and cared about such things—yet he insisted I was the most beautiful woman he had ever known."[131] If new surgical procedures hold for the post-mastectomy woman the promise of "very pretty boobies," it is important to recognize that this is a promise clearly linked with the promise of attractiveness to others (especially men). This promise makes concrete the heterosexist paradigm in which this narrative operates and is exemplified by Queller's discussions of her post-mastectomy boyfriend.

The second theme that emerges related to transforming women's bodies is the promise of the better self with better breasts. For Queller, the better breasts are smaller breasts: "I launched into my speech about how I wanted smaller breasts, how all these years of being a D-cup had driven me crazy."[132] The mastectomy and reconstruction process had what Queller calls "guilty pleasures," including the ability to choose a new breast size.[133] Applegate jokes about similar issues: "You know, I'm gonna have cute boobs 'til I'm ninety, so, you know, there's that. I'm gonna have the best boobs in the nursing home. I'm telling you. I'm gonna be the envy of all the ladies around the bridge table."[134] In the same light tone, she tells Oprah, "I don't have to wear a bra!"[135] Better breasts in both discussions are those that mirror more perfectly society's definition of beautiful breasts: whether large or small, the breasts described here are perky. These are not breasts that will sag with time or that will ever need the support of a bra. In many ways, these are not breasts that can be found in nature. However, they are presented here as better than natural breasts.

More important than simply having better breasts, however, is the sense that with the better breasts comes a better, truer self. Carl Elliott suggests that people engaging in various forms of technological self-transformation, from body building to sex-reassignment surgery, tend to experience this not as the creation of a new self but the discovery of a more authentic true self and therefore as a project of self-realization, of becoming who they really are.[136] Queller's narrative of self-realization demonstrates how the process of having a prophylactic mastectomy brought her closer to her real self. Throughout her memoir Queller explains how her breasts are important to her identity. She had large breasts like her mother and sister, labeled herself (and was labeled by others) a "buxom Jewess," and was ultimately uncomfortable in her own body and very ambivalent about her breasts. Her body was not a reflection of who she really was: "Somewhere along the line I'd started equating my big boobs with the bimbo persona I so loathed. I had a love-hate relationship with my breasts. I did not want to be valued for them."[137] Nevertheless, Queller recognizes that her breasts are important to the extent that she partakes in a "goodbye ceremony" to her breasts that included two photo sessions with friends and a professional photographer. Similarly, Applegate also had her "first and last nudie photo shoot" at her home, including what she describes as close-ups from every angle, "so I can remember them."[138] The centrality of breasts to women's identity has been well documented, and in an interview study with women who underwent prophylactic mastectomies, Nina Hallowell notes that "they [her participants] described their femininity as being dependent upon maintaining a particular body shape—having breasts. Mastectomy was, therefore, viewed as a threat to their femininity in so far as it results in a deficient body—a body that is no longer feminine."[139] However, in striking contrast to the women Hallowell interviewed, the prophylactic mastectomy narrative represents the post-mastectomy, post-reconstruction woman as more, not less, feminine than before. In Queller's case, the mastectomy and her reconstructed breasts allow her to close the gap between her identity and her body: "I feel completely comfortable and at home in my new body."[140]

Applegate enacts a similar feeling of comfort in her new body in various post-mastectomy interviews and appearances that reaffirm her movie-star beauty. First known for playing the not-so-bright teenager Kelly Bundy in the 1980s hit sitcom *Married . . . with Children*, Applegate's characters and her appearance matured in the 1990s.[141] At the time of her diagnosis with breast cancer, Applegate was playing the vivacious and beautiful Samantha on another hit sitcom, *Samantha Who?* Walking onto the *Oprah* set in a tight black skirt, high heels, and a form-fitting green top (revealing the curve of her reconstructed breasts), Applegate is stunning, and Winfrey draws attention to her beauty with her opening statement: "You look great."[142] Oprah confirms that Applegate's career of playing beautiful blondes is in no way threatened by her double mastectomy. An article in *People* discussed in detail Applegate's form-fitting one-shouldered blue dress at the 2008 Emmy awards (complementing her "red carpet glow"), and the magazine put Applegate on their Emmy Awards best-dressed list.[143] Celebrity gossip web site *Popsugar* captured the overall feeling regarding Applegate's appearance: "Christina Applegate looked positively radiant and was the talk of the night—smiley, happy and healthy."[144] Applegate emerges from her cancer crisis and her double mastectomy with rave reviews from the press that not only confirm Applegate's continued status as a Hollywood beauty but also suggest that her beauty is even greater than it was before her cancer experience. In the words of the reviews of Applegate's Emmy appearance, she is radiant, glowing, and happy.

Hallowell suggests that "the practice of maintaining or managing the properly feminine body has implications for self, in the sense that managing the body entails managing the self."[145] Queller's new body reflects her true self (a serious writer instead of a bimbo) and also reflects the ongoing management— and transformation—of the body required by women in postfeminist culture. The downside of Queller's and Applegate's transformations is perhaps best explained by Sue Tait, who decries the postfeminist logic in which "a celebration of the body, the pleasure of transformation, and individual empowerment function [as] a justification for a renewed objectification of female bodies."[146] The identity of the cancer/risk-free woman articulated in this discourse— one that is fleshed out in the detailed descriptions of breasts and breast reconstructions—is inhabitable by only a small segment of society (white, wealthy, heterosexual) and continues to closely relate breasts with feminine identity. In a striking fashion, the choice to have a prophylactic double mastectomy becomes part of what Tasker and Negra describe as the "aggressive mainstreaming of elaborate and expensive beauty treatments to the middle class," a process that perpetuates an image of woman as pinup.[147] As represented in this narrative, a young woman can potentially emerge from the process of having a double prophylactic mastectomy and reconstructive surgery feeling more at home in her body than she had before, both because she has successfully removed the risk of breast cancer from her life and because the surgeries offered her a chance to realign her body to reflect her true self.

Compulsory Choice and Biomedical Subjects

The prophylactic mastectomy narrative demonstrates the alignment of genetic risk with larger neoliberal constructions of risk. Specifically, individual responsibility for one's health and an emphasis on individual agency—one's ability to make choices—are the central aspects of the discourse about prophylactic

mastectomies. However, the method of empowerment through choice offered
in this narrative—whether or not to have a prophylactic mastectomy—is not a
choice at all. The roughly 87 percent lifetime risk of breast cancer for women
who are BRCA positive (the percentage given by Queller) is framed in the
narrative as an unacceptable risk. For the many women who have watched a
family member struggle with cancer, cancer is understandably not a risk to be
entertained. What the prophylactic mastectomy narrative makes clear is the
very power of risk calculations. Although I argue that we should question the
presentation of risks regarding health issues, from the emphasis on some risk
factors over others to the very complex nature of statistical measures, the vulnerable empowered women of this narrative do not have the space to question
risk. Once vulnerability to cancer is framed as unacceptable, the vulnerable
empowered woman's choices are placed in a highly moralized context with
a focus on the possibilities of a better self, a context that offers prophylactic
mastectomies as a compulsory choice for women with BRCA gene mutations.
Strengthening this sense of compulsory action is a reliance on a postfeminist
logic that promises women empowerment (by, for example, ridding themselves
of the risk of cancer) but justifies that empowerment through traditional gendered configurations of home and family. The identity of the cancer/risk-free
woman is thoroughly ensconced within traditional expectations for women
about both motherhood and heterosexual partnerships.

The focus on issues of reproduction and sexuality in the prophylactic
mastectomy narrative are not unexpected. Breast cancer threatens a woman's
sexual functioning and ability to have children or take care of those she already
has. What makes the prophylactic mastectomy narrative of mainstream public
discourse worrisome is how these issues are framed. As they are constructed
through a heterosexual paradigm, for example, the problems of breast cancer
and relationships are reduced to finding and/or keeping the perfect man. The
lived experiences of BRCA-positive lesbians—who are also concerned with
their children and are also concerned about their relationships—do not meld
easily with the expectations of public discourse. The lack of visibility of lesbian
women in breast cancer culture has a long history. As just one example, sitting
in the hospital after her mastectomy in 1978, Audre Lorde finishes a conversation with a well-meaning Reach for Recovery volunteer who was promising
her that men would still find her attractive by thinking to herself, "I wonder if
there are any black lesbian feminists in Reach for Recovery?"[148] Many women
in positions dramatically different from those of Applegate or Queller—
lesbians, working-class women, African American women, older women, and

so forth—may opt for prophylactic surgery for reasons that do not align with the prophylactic mastectomy narrative. The exclusion of these varying experiences smoothes over the complexity of the breast cancer experience in favor of an identity that is clearly aligned with both postfeminist and neoliberal forces.

The problems of the identity of the cancer/risk-free woman—the compulsory acceptance of a contested procedure and the reification of traditional femininity—are also a part of a larger dynamic of the prophylactic mastectomy narrative: the deepening of the division between women who exist within and those who exist outside of the biomedical establishment. The cancer/risk-free subjectivity is not just embedded within hegemonic discourses of femininity and sexuality but also within discourses of race and class. Although Queller recognizes that new genetic tests are "not without their perils," she ends her memoir with a clear call for women to "seize" new scientific advances.[149] As the exemplar of the cancer/risk-free woman, Queller enacts this seizing: she endures numerous tests and visits to doctors, three surgeries, and three unsuccessful rounds of in vitro fertilization. What goes unsaid—but remains highly visible—in Queller's story is her privilege. Queller, Applegate, Linder, and the many other representatives of prophylactic mastectomies had unparalleled access to biomedicine and the medical establishment that other women simply do not share.

In her discussion of the regime of biomedicalization in breast cancer culture, Maren Klawiter suggests that it is unique in its ability to transform what had been a temporary role of a person with an illness for some women (in the early and mid-twentieth century, women were diagnosed, treated, and declared "cured") to a permanent "risk role" for all women—a role that entails constant surveillance and medical supervision.[150] By the late twentieth century (coinciding with the rise of survivor culture) all women could be placed somewhere on the breast cancer continuum: as low or high risk, in remission or not yet diagnosed, and so forth. The development of a cancer/risk-free identity, however, shifts the risk role for women in at least one significant way. Privileged women who already have access to the extensive medical treatment can, for the first time, attempt to opt out of the permanent risk role by making themselves cancer/risk-free. However, this option does not entirely rid them of their risk (although it is often presented as if it does), and it requires an intense entrenchment within medical culture. The cancer/risk-free woman is not released from breast cancer culture; rather, she signals the solidification of biomedical empowerment as the primary means through which cancer can be prevented. This solidification of biomedical empowerment is particularly important because it leaves little space for discussing other means of preventing cancer, including reducing environmental toxins, which would necessitate large-scale social—not merely individual—action.

Empowerment through biomedicine is not necessarily (or essentially) negative. Indeed, women's active involvement in biomedical culture, and (as represented through the prophylactic mastectomy narrative) their empowerment through biomedical culture is part of the era of biomedicalization in which, as Rose writes, we have "growing capacities to control, manage, engineer, reshape, and modulate the very vital capacities of human beings as living creatures."[151] Rather than share the distrust of many critics, Rose insists that "instead I argue that we are seeing the emergence of a novel somatic ethics, imposing obligations yet imbued with hope, oriented to the future yet demanding action in the present."[152] Prophylactic mastectomies do hold out hope to women; by acting in the present, women are represented as securing a cancer/risk-free future. My concern with women's empowerment through entrenchment within biomedical culture is based on how women's choices are represented and thus how those choices are made sense of in connection to issues of gender, sexuality, race, and class. The choice of prophylactic mastectomies is represented as occurring within a relational context that is embedded in the heterosexual matrix, or the "naturalized and reified notions of gender that support masculine hegemony and heterosexist power."[153] While women's lived experiences may include a wider variety of lifestyles and issues that factor into their decisions, this variety is reduced in dominant public discourse to one issue: the need to secure, or maintain, a traditional nuclear family. In terms of gender, the representational politics of prophylactic mastectomies are problematic because they not only offer up an identity (and a means of empowerment) that ties women's personhood to children and husbands but they also reaffirm for the larger audience a very traditional understanding of gender roles and relations.

The class and race privilege of the empowered biomedical citizen, here represented by the cancer/risk-free woman, also points to another significant problem with reducing women's opportunities of empowerment to biomedical answers. Nikolas Rose recognizes the problem of privilege on an international scale, noting that the field of biomedicine operates in "two parallel universes" in which the developed world is positioned to take advantage of new biotechnological advances and the "underdeveloped world" continues to suffer from basic health problems caused by extreme poverty.[154] In the prophylactic mastectomy narrative, the parallel universes of empowered and disempowered are represented through the empowered figure of the cancer/risk-free woman and an invisible disempowered figure. These disempowered individuals—who because of material and cultural inequalities related to race, class, gender, sexuality, and so forth—do not have the ability to visit countless doctors, undergo medical procedures not covered by health insurance, and reconstruct their bodies and identities. These individuals are both disempowered and at risk for the diseases that more privileged individuals have avoided. And these individuals are all but invisible in public discourse about breast cancer. For disempowered and at-risk women, the permanent risk role identified by Klawiter as part of the biomedical regime becomes even more fraught with problems, as they are not only permanently at risk but they also lack access to resources to fulfill their own responsibility for ensuring their health and well-being.

As just one example of the contemporary postfeminist public discourse about women's health, the prophylactic mastectomy narrative should prompt numerous questions and concerns about how women are being situated in relation to their bodies and the larger medical industry. The prophylactic mastectomy narrative also raises the question of what might be different if a feminist perspective were more available. Although I discuss what a feminist perspective on women's health in the twenty-first century might look like in the final chapter, two points can be made now. First, one area in which feminist activists have already taken action is on the issue of gene patents. In 2009, Breast Cancer Action joined the American Civil Liberties Union and a coalition of women's health organizations, scientific organizations, and individual women to challenge the legality of gene patents. The BCA web site explains, "We believe it's wrong for the government to give one company the power to dictate all scientific and medical uses of genes that each of us has in our bodies. We urgently need more and better options for the treatment and risk reduction of breast cancer, and we cannot afford to have progress stymied by the monopolies that gene patents create."[155] Myriad Genetic Laboratories' patent on the BRCA1 and BRCA2 mutations meant that it held all rights to not only the genes but also to any genetic testing associated with the genes. Patenting genes is a salient example of privilege because "Myriad's monopoly on the BRCA genes allows it to set the price for a full sequencing test—currently over $3,000. Many qualified geneticists could do the testing for less but cannot because of the patents. Women who do not have insurance that covers the test and who cannot afford Myriad's price are denied the ability to make informed medical decisions."[156] In March 2010, a New York district court struck down the patent, arguing that "the identification of the BRCA1 and BRCA2 gene sequences is unquestionably a valuable scientific achievement for which Myriad deserves recognition, but that is not the same as concluding that it is something for which they are entitled to patent."[157] Although Myriad is appealing the ruling, the success of the lawsuit points to the courts as one viable avenue of feminist action.

Second, BCA is on record as the only national breast cancer organization to join the lawsuit, a stance made possible because of their independence from corporations, pharmaceutical companies, and other biomedical organizations.[158] By refusing sponsorship by the biomedical industry, BCA is positioned as an outsider organization that sees both the promise and the problems of biomedicalization. Amanda Schaffer, a blogger for Double X (a feminist blog attached to the left-leaning online magazine *Slate*), attempts to articulate a similar stance through her own personal narrative.[159] Schaffer questions the dominant narrative in which women are applauded for having prophylactic mastectomies, although she does recognize that women's choices about mastectomies may be in reaction to the downsides of lumpectomies: the follow-up chemotherapy and radiation, the fearful years of mammograms, and the overall uncertainty. What is striking about the picture that Schaffer paints, however, is its embrace of uncertainty and the gray areas of cancer treatments and decisions. Treatments are all double-edged swords in Schaffer's narrative, and after recalling the years of the Halsted radical mastectomy and the feminist protests against mastectomies, Schaffer concludes that "it is hard not to worry that more women than need to are choosing to cut off their breasts."[160] Schaffer offers no specific answers to the problem of prophylactic mastectomies, but her perspective includes the room to question the treatment, medical experts, and dominant breast cancer culture. Indeed, many writers and bloggers such as Schaffer are working to provide the discursive space in which challenging medical authorities and questioning treatments from a feminist perspective is routine.

Chapter 3

Postfeminist Risky Mothers and Postpartum Depression

In her landmark 1976 book *Of Woman Born: Motherhood as Experience and Institution*, Adrienne Rich describes motherhood as an institution that works— through a series of organizational structures and cultural belief systems—to restrain women's agency by reducing their lives to the domestic sphere. The institution of motherhood ensures that women's potential relationship with the "powers of reproduction" remains "under male control."[1] Rich writes, "It [the institution] has withheld over one-half the human species from the decisions affecting their lives; it exonerates men from fatherhood in any authentic sense; it creates the dangerous schism between 'private' and 'public' life; it calcifies human choices and potentialities."[2] Rich makes sure to separate the institution of motherhood from the practice of bearing and caring for children; the institution creates "prescriptions and conditions in which choices are made or blocked."[3] An important part of what makes the institution of motherhood powerful is cultural beliefs about what makes a good mother. Variously described as myths or ideologies, discourses about good mothers construct a specific set of expectations. Rich, for example, describes the concept of the "natural mother," one who "is a person without further identity, one who can find her chief gratification in being all day with small children, living at a pace tuned to theirs" and who experiences maternal love as "literally selfless."[4]

Contemporary discourses of good motherhood do not exist in a cultural vacuum. As Angela Davis argues, "The historical construction of women's reproductive role, which is largely synonymous with the historical failure to acknowledge the possibility of reproductive self-determination, has been informed by a peculiar constellation of racist and misogynist assumptions."[5] Good motherhood is raced and classed: white, upper-middle-class, heterosexual women's experiences are routinely privileged over those of working-class women or women of color. In the late twentieth century, the concerns of white, privileged mothers—the incessant anxiety about fertility and access to reproductive technologies, the consumerism, and the constructed mommy wars between stay-at-home and working mothers—made up the background for the expectations of good motherhood. Bad mothers were routinely represented in popular culture through a series of images and anecdotes that drew heavily on narratives about race and class: the crack mother and her crack baby, the welfare mother, and the teenage mother. While mothering in the shadow of cultural expectations for the good mother is a difficult task for all women (even the women most clearly constructed as the audience for the discourse of good motherhood—white, privileged, heterosexual women—routinely fail), for women who are "othered," good mothering will always remain out of reach.

Although women enact mothering in concert with expectations about what it means to be a good mother that have changed over time, in the overarching myth of the good mother, certain expectations stay the same. Roderick Hart defines myths as "master stories describing exceptional people doing exceptional things and serving as moral guides to proper action."[6] Three of the hallmarks of the myth of the good mother are women's instinctual ability to nurture their children (although definitions of good nurturing may change from decade to decade), women's selflessness in relation to their children, and a child-centered approach that places the well-being and happiness of children above all other issues. The myth of the good mother depends on the construction of a bad mother. Without a recognizable bad mother, good mothers, as Susan Douglas and Meredith Michaels wryly note, have no one to revile, no one to look to as a means of reassurance of one's own status as a good mother.[7] Feminist responses to the myth of the good mother have been diverse. The goals of second-wave feminists regarding motherhood included the "rejection of technology, the search for 'authentic experience,' the prizing of youth and innocence, the revalorization of nature, the reclamation of the body and reinscription of sexuality, and the search for community" but generally were united in their attempt to point to the constructed nature of good motherhood and how the myth of good motherhood shapes actual mothering practices.[8] The variety of responses has not been easy to parse out in public culture, and one of the stereotypes feminists continue to face is that they (at best) ignore motherhood and mothers or (at worst) are against motherhood and mothers. Whether feminists respond to the constraints of good mothering by suggesting, like Adrienne Rich, that patriarchy has alienated women from the potential their procreative capacity endows them with or by insisting, like Ti Grace Atkinson, upon the "true, brutal nature" of motherhood, feminists theorists and activists have long approached mothering from a critical standpoint that enables them to offer critiques of the myth of good motherhood and replace the myth with their own theories of motherhood.[9]

I have begun this chapter with a discussion of the myth of good motherhood and feminist responses to the social construction of mothering because I see constructions of mothering as a pivotal part of public discussions about postpartum disorders. I am not alone in this claim; as Barbara Barnett, a journalism scholar, has so amply demonstrated in her analysis of the case of Andrea Yates, who drowned her five children in 2001 and was represented in the media as suffering from postpartum psychosis, Yates was presented as a good mother gone either mad or bad in most press coverage.[10] In this chapter, I analyze two best-selling memoirs about postpartum depression, Brooke Shields's *Down Came the Rain: My Journey Through Postpartum Depression* and Heather Armstrong's *It Sucked and Then I Cried: How I Had a Baby, a Breakdown, and a Much Needed Margarita*, and selected mommy blogs and news coverage of postpartum disorders during the period 2005 to 2010.[11] I suggest that the memoirs, blogs, and news coverage participate in constructing a relatively new version of the myth of good motherhood: the postfeminist narrative of risky motherhood. Like feminist critiques of the myth of good motherhood, this new narrative appears to insist that mothering is often difficult and push back against expectations of perfection and the assumption that all women have an innate maternal instinct. Even so, postfeminist risky mothers align themselves with the mythical good mother by replicating several key facets of the myth of good motherhood. Second, I argue that the narrative of risky motherhood normalizes postpartum depression through the identity of the *risky mother*. First, however, I turn to a brief discussion of the history behind the tension between biomedical definitions of postpartum disorders and understandings of postpartum disorders that emphasize the lived context of mothering.

Postpartum Disorders and the Struggles of Motherhood

What we now frequently refer to as postpartum disorders have a long history. By the nineteenth century, what was known as "puerperal insanity" accounted for about 10 percent of asylum admissions.[12] The symptoms of this "disease" that were identified at the time were notable for their anti-feminine qualities:

using obscenity, aversion to the child and the husband, and meanness, to name a few.[13] In perhaps the most famous depiction of emotional turbulence during the postpartum period, Charlotte Perkins Gilman's *The Yellow Wallpaper* (1892) tells the story of a woman who feels trapped by her role as wife and mother and is further incapacitated by the medical treatment she receives. One interpretation of women's distress during the postpartum period, as Gilman's work suggests, is that it is a response (even a resistance) to the oppressive dimensions of being a mother. Verta Taylor suggests that during the postpartum period women feel "desperation and rebellion against maternal constraints."[14] Such an interpretation emphasizes the social aspects of our emotions and configures women's distress as related to their social environment and not necessarily their physiological processes. However, postpartum distress is now almost universally understood as a mental illness, and the medicalization of postpartum disorders today is being propelled at least in part by women.[15]

Postpartum mood disorders—a broad spectrum of recognized mental health disorders that includes depression, anxiety, obsessive-compulsive disorder, and psychosis—are now situated squarely within disciplines of psychiatry, psychology, and related fields that have long been the subjects of critiques by feminist scholars. Women's health activists associated with the second wave, for example, recognized that psychiatric discourses "recast women's responses to subordination as disorder, hysteria, or madness."[16] More recently, critics such as Linda Blum and Nena Stracuzzi have argued that psychiatric diagnoses rest more on cultural biases than on physiological evidence: "Mental illness is not only gendered in biomedical terms, with disproportionate cases of particular disorders among male or female individuals; mental illness is also constructed and understood in terms that convey femininity or masculinity, that produce and police their boundaries."[17] Because of psychiatry's inability to demonstrate organic correlates of its diagnoses, the field was easily positioned by feminist critics as producing "diagnoses [that] merely medicalized deviance and upheld the norms of a patriarchal social order."[18] However, since the 1990s, psychiatry and psychology have turned to increasingly sophisticated technology that has literally reduced the "mind" (our thoughts and emotional landscapes) into the systems of the brain. This transformation—from understanding emotional landscapes as part of a broad psychological space to mapping them upon the brain itself—plays an important role in contemporary psychiatric explanations for postpartum disorders.

The fourth edition of the *Diagnostic and Statistical Manual of Mental Disorders* (DSM) officially recognized postpartum depression in 1994, offering for clinicians the specifier "with postpartum onset" for major depressive disorder if the depression occurred within four weeks of giving birth of a child.[19] Practicing physicians have extended the time of onset to the first full year after childbirth.[20] Although definitions and statistics vary, most medical researchers agree that postpartum disorders exist on a continuum (the "baby blues," postpartum depression, and postpartum psychosis) and constitute serious mental health problems. As Michael O'Hara explains, "Postpartum depression should be distinguished from the postpartum blues, which refers to mood symptoms that are common in the first week to 10 days after delivery and usually resolve within a few days without any intervention. Symptoms include mood lability, irritability, interpersonal hypersensitivity, insomnia, anxiety, tearfulness, and sometimes elation. . . . At the other end of the spectrum is postpartum psychosis, which is characterized by severely depressed mood, disorganized thinking, psychotic thoughts, and hallucinations."[21] O'Hara's definitions are derived from the standard understanding of the symptoms of postpartum depression. He notes that as many as 7.1 percent of women may suffer from a major depressive episode within three months after giving birth.[22] This number increases to 19.2 percent if women with minor depression are included. Postpartum psychosis, on the other hand, is far more rare, affecting only 0.1 to 0.2 percent of women in the general population.[23]

The psychiatric literature on postpartum disorders is characterized by a search for and emphasis on the possible physiological factors that cause postpartum disorders. Uriel Halbreich, for example, suggests that postpartum mood disorders such as postpartum depression belong in a broader class of mood disorders related to women's reproductive functions: "Reproductive Related Disorders (RRDs) in women are a group of interdisciplinary diagnostic entities characterized by their timing—that is linked to reproductive processes, diversified phenomenology, epidemiological associations, and shared vulnerabilities."[24] What ties RRDs together—the shared vulnerability, a particularly interesting phrase given my interest in the vulnerable woman—is hormones. Halbreich suggests that there are two important components of the pathophysiology of RRDs: a genetic vulnerability shaped by life episodes and worsened by hormonal changes and maladaptation to hormonal withdrawal or instability.[25] That hormones are the culprit should not be a surprise—women's health research has long focused (often inaccurately) on women's hormones as the root of all sickness.[26] What is different about Halbreich's argument—which was published in 2010—is the new ascension of genetics. Like the research on breast cancer, research on postpartum disorders has begun to look for genetic vulnerabilities.

The changing psychiatric gaze, from a moral gaze (medicalizing deviance, for example) to a molecular gaze that classifies disorders through a language of neurotransmitters and treats them through psychiatric drugs, has specific implications for the treatment of individuals with "faulty neuro-processes."[27] The most prominent flaw in such treatment regimens, according to feminist psychologists, is a lack of attention to the power structures and cultural institutions that may play a role in the development of certain disorders. Working from outside a strictly biomedical paradigm, feminist psychologists have long offered nonbiological explanations for women's mental illness, and certainly for postpartum depression. Psychologist Paula Nicolson's woman-centered approach to postpartum depression, for example, points to the idea of loss—namely, loss of identity, loss of a past life with activities and friends, loss of autonomy, loss of time—as one of the many social factors that constitute the etiology of postpartum depression.[28] Psychologists—even those that may not self-identify as feminist—are more inclined to include social factors as part of any discussion of the multiple factors that might cause a case of postpartum depression. Feminists link many of these factors—such as marital unhappiness, poor birth experiences, and low social support—to larger patriarchal systems, as these factors are (to use Laura Brown's phrase) "discomforts of the powerless."[29]

The tension between feminist/psychological explanations of postpartum disorders that focus largely on the social context and molecular/psychiatric explanations has not been easily resolved, and the history of the postpartum depression self-help movement partially explains why. Verta Taylor's nuanced analysis of the self-help movement focuses on two groups, Postpartum Support International (PSI) and Depression After Delivery (DAD), both of which were formed by women who had experienced debilitating mental illness after birth but were unable to find sources of treatment and support.[30] Like feminist psychologists, women who participate in postpartum self-help groups often look to the social context of postpartum depression. Jane Honikman, the founder of PSI, organized her first support group around a "feminist frame that linked maternal depression to the sexual division of labor in the family that gives women primary responsibility for rearing and nurturing children but places them at a distinct disadvantage in the public world."[31] With cultural expectations for motherhood suggesting that women should be joyful, happy, instantly in love with their new babies, and at peace with their new identity of mom, the women interviewed by Taylor struggled with experiences that did not meet cultural expectations for good mothering. Women felt guilty for not feeling an intense "mother love" with their new infants, anxiety and fear about handling the baby properly, and significant depression when they discussed the loss of self that comes with being a mother.[32]

Unfortunately, looking to cultural expectations for mothers as an explanation for postpartum mood disorders does not offer easy ways of helping women who are experiencing postpartum distress. Laura Brown captures the problem: "Practicing feminist-informed psychotherapists have been confronted with the reality of suffering human beings seeking care to ameliorate their distress. These individuals frequently must be given a formal diagnosis of a disorder to gain access to or payment for services."[33] Not only is a formal diagnosis important for access to services, it also plays a pivotal role in women's self-acceptance. Having a diagnosis removes the stigma from the deviant emotions mothers experience after birth. Instead of living with a stigma, women are asked to live with—and treat—a medically identifiable disease. For this reason, postpartum self-help groups have played an important role in the institutionalization and indeed in the medicalization of postpartum depression. They were pivotal, for example, in advocating for the inclusion of the "with postpartum onset" specifier in the 1994 DSM. The process of medicalization has long been demonized by feminist critics who have argued that medicine has overstepped its authority by pulling aspects of women's lives into the medical sphere.[34] Medicalization is linked in such criticism with pathologization.[35] However, the postpartum depression self-help movement showcases what Rose describes as the inescapable influence of medicine: "We relate to ourselves and others, individually and collectively, through an ethic and in a form of life that is inextricably associated with medicine in all of its incarnations."[36] Without a medical diagnosis, mainstream recognition of what we now call postpartum depression would be difficult. Advocating for recognition of postpartum depression as a disease may seem counterintuitive in light of feminist critiques of the process of medicalization, but most postpartum self-help advocates walk the careful line between recognizing the physiological effects (and possible causes) of postpartum disorders and at the same time emphasizing the need to address the social context of postpartum distress: motherhood.

This type of advocacy has been relatively successful in terms of prompting doctors and researchers to pay attention to the postpartum period. In the late 1980s and throughout the 1990s, postpartum disorders received both more media and medical attention than they had in the previous decades. Nationally recognized academic hospitals—such as the Ohio State University Hospital—have created postpartum clinics in response to lobbying by activists.[37] However, the balance between "contextual" and "biological" all too often sways public understandings of postpartum disorders toward the bio-medical viewpoint. Renee Martinez, Ingrid Johnston-Robledo, Heather Ulsh, and Joan Chrisler report in their analysis of magazine coverage of postpartum disorders from 1980 to 1998 that "the majority of the articles we examined pro-moted the medical model"; 68 percent of the articles on postpartum depression mentioned hormones as a cause.[38] Often missing were discussions of the fac-tors about motherhood that might make a woman distressed: "The articles that focused on hormones as the cause of postpartum affective disturbances rarely mentioned other reasons why women might feel sad or irritable immediately after giving birth, such as recovery from a painful and exhausting labor and birth, disappointment that the process of labor and birth was not as expected, fatigue, problems with breast feeding, or the stress of being 'on call' 24 hours a day."[39] These factors are absolutely essential in understanding the development of what we understand as postpartum disorders. More broadly, I suggest that our constructions of motherhood are instrumental in shaping how we under-stand both postpartum disorders and women who suffer from them.

In the analysis that follows I point to how one particular construction of good motherhood works to normalize postpartum depression by articulating women as risky mothers. I continue throughout this case study to discuss moth-ers using the language of postpartum disorders and/or postpartum depression, but I should emphasize that I recognize "postpartum depression" and other similar terms as labels that were constructed in psychiatric discourse to cat-egorize a particular group of emotions and behaviors. In my use of these labels, I hope to avoid confusion about the experiences I am discussing (namely, the emotional turbulence some women feel after the birth of a child), but I am not signaling an unquestioning endorsement of the medicalization of those experiences.

The Risky Motherhood Narrative and the Postfeminist Risky Mother

According to *New York Times* writer David Hochman, "The world's most thank-less occupation, parenthood, has never inspired so much copy."[40] Although Hochman focuses on parenting broadly—his article includes a discussion of fathering blogs—considerations of postfeminist motherhood have dominated the blogosphere, popular fiction ("mommy lit" is a recognized subgenre of "chick lit"), and entertainment media (examples include Uma Thurman's 2010 movie *Motherhood*).[41] In what follows, I examine how mommy blogs and Brooke Shields's and Heather Armstrong's postpartum depression memoirs take part in the construction of a larger cultural narrative of risky motherhood. Although the narrative of risky motherhood is often positioned as a refutation of the myth of good motherhood, two dynamics in these texts suggest that women who participate in the narrative of risky motherhood are a postfeminist iteration of good mothers: the shifting definitions of good and bad mothering and the assertion of love for children.

The narrative of risky mothering in popular culture asserts that mothers face challenges in their daily lives: a woman who becomes a mother faces dramatic identity changes, may feel resentful about her new duties as a primary caregiver, and at times makes mistakes. Rather than feeling shame at their fallibility, however, mothers in the narrative of risky motherhood embrace it: "Over coffee and out in cyberspace they are gleefully labeling themselves 'bad mommies,' pouring out their doubts, their dissatisfaction and their dysfunction, celebrating their own shortcomings in contrast to their older sisters' cloying perfection."[42] In the face of cultural assumptions and expectations that align with the myth of the good mother, the label "bad mommies" is particularly significant. It is not a claiming of the bad mother as constructed in the myth of good motherhood (remembering of course that bad mothers are often women of color, poor women, drug-addicted women, and so forth) but rather a demarcation of what is acceptably bad as opposed to unacceptably bad. One blogger explains the distinction: "I've learnt that being a 'bad mommy' doesn't mean you don't care. Or that you're really a bad person. Sometimes it's what your kid needs. Letting them drink the bathwater, eat grass, and suck the carpet is not the end of the world."[43] Bad mommies are not bad people, she notes, but rather are mothers who are pragmatic and expedient. Thus, unlike the models of perfection in the myth of good motherhood, mothers in the narrative of risky motherhood are represented as engaging in imperfect behavior, often including risky behaviors, such as letting a child eat grass.

Mothers in the risky motherhood narrative—from Brooke Shields and Heather Armstrong to the hundreds of mommy bloggers—are frank in their assessment of their abilities and fallibilities. The author of "A Bad Mommy Blog" offers a description of what she calls "real moms"; her list includes several items that point directly to the function of risky mothers as being able to distinguish between the myth of good motherhood and the "reality" of motherhood. Real moms "do not mince words when they present the truth," "know that real life is not like TV sitcoms," and "aren't afraid to dish the dirt on motherhood."[44] In the narrative of risky motherhood, bad mommy moments are often those moments when reality collides with expectations. Many of these

collisions happen when women fail to meet cultural expectations that mothers should be selfless. Heather Armstrong, for example, describes the joy of
spending her first weekend away from her daughter on a romantic trip with her
husband: "We indulged in room service and then got sushi and then ordered
champagne at 1PM in the afternoon for brunch. We ran naked to the hot tub
and sat in front of the fireplace to dry off."[45] One blogging mother describes her
negotiation with her child, who wanted help to find her lost goggles, through
the instructions given by most airlines: "In case of an emergency, please remember to secure your own oxygen mask first."[46] She constructs the moment for her
readers, "I speak around my toothbrush, 'I said that I am dealing with my own
emergency first. I am brushing my teeth and brushing my hair and rinsing my
face. Once I am all calm and settled and oxygen is flowing freely through my
mask? Then I will come down to deal with your goggles emergency.'"[47] The bad
mommy moments in the narrative of risky motherhood are moments of failure
(whether deliberate or not) when placed next to the mythical good mother. But,
as in the case of the mother facing the goggle emergency, bad mommy moments
are mundane. Although they embrace the label of bad mommy, the mothers in
the narrative of risky motherhood are secure in the position of good motherhood, both through the relative harmlessness of their "badness" and through
their reaffirmation of one of the central aspects of good mothering: devotion to
and love for their children.

As the women who practice risky motherhood describe their everyday
experiences, they are clearly full of a variety of emotions, including emotions
that we often understand as negative such as frustration, sadness, anger, and
anxiety. One blogger, Domestic Diva, describes her situation this way: "I went
to bed one night a fit and fabulous 25 year old bride, and woke up one day a
flabby and frazzled 32 year old mother of three."[48] The frazzled mom explains
her everyday life with a bit of wryness, "Honestly though, most days it's a victory if I manage to brush my own teeth by noon. I also find my new 'Domestic'
situation requires a large amount of patience and an equal amount of humor.
Most days, if I wasn't laughing, I'd be crying."[49] What makes the ups and downs
of motherhood—the frazzled state, the flabbiness—worthwhile is the mother's
love for her children. Throughout the mommy blogs, readers are reminded time
and again of the one underlying emotion that makes the moms' work worthwhile: love. Mrs. Foreste describes her feelings about being a stay-at-home mom
(SAHM): "I love being a full time SAHM more than anything, as I've said many
times before. . . . All I have to do is look at that smil[e]y face of Gianna's when
she discovers she's able to do something new & I know I made the right decision

with the 'job' I chose."[50] The brief reference to Gianna's face and "knowing" that she's made the right decision to stay home stands in for a larger, more explicit discussion of love. This more explicit discussion is abundantly apparent in other blogs and certainly in both of the postpartum memoirs. The woman who blogs Becoming Sarah describes taking a nap with her daughter: "THIS, I find myself thinking as we wake up peering into one another's eyes, this is love. This, right here, right now, this moment. This is the greatest love that ever was, that ever will be."[51] Brooke Shields also writes at length on the subject of loving her daughter, explaining, "Holding Rowan, I felt special and needed. I realized there was an undeniable bond between my little girl and me. It couldn't be usurped by anything or anyone. This was unique and it was ours."[52] The declarations of love and the framing of motherhood as a life-changing experience (for the better) soften the negligible bad mommy moments. That is, although a mom might watch her child fall on the playground or might fail at making homemade cookies for her daughter's birthday party, her endless, bountiful love ensures that everything will work out.

Although the mothers I have discussed are represented as unified in their dedication to a more pragmatic view of mothering—to a tolerance of the risks of mothering that come with their own imperfections—that contrasts starkly with the myth of the good mother, they are equally devoted to declaring their love for their children. This love places children at the center of their lives, even when they are determined to find space for themselves. For despite their fallibility, these mothers are still good mothers (that is, they align with the core values of the myth of the good mother despite their at-times explicit rejection of the myth). Recognizing this, the subtitle of the Her Bad Mother blog is Bad Is the New Good.[53] The narrative of risky motherhood is simply a postfeminist iteration of good motherhood in which a limited number of fallibilities are accepted as long as mothers continue to demonstrate love for—and substantial self-definition through—their children.

The contemporary narrative of risky motherhood follows a particular pattern: mothers declare their imperfections (often through the label bad mommy) as opposed to allegiance with the mythical good mother but return in the end to a trope of love and fulfillment through their children that realigns them with the myth of good mother. The protagonists of this narrative—mothers who claim their imperfections—are best understood as postfeminist risky mothers. This identity, like theories of the maternal instinct, suggests that women are inherently (biologically) nurturers, but even as an instinctual nurturer, the postfeminist risky mother is not perfect. She engages in mothering practices that may not be the best for her children and she feels emotions other than joy and happiness about mothering. These imperfections are accepted—they are part of the reality of risky mothering—but they nonetheless position the mother as risky in terms of her ongoing ability to protect and serve her children.

As I suggested in my analysis of the discourse surrounding prophylactic mastectomies, postfeminist depictions of women's health tend to focus on white, upper-middle-class, heterosexual women. This elite club is also the focus of the hegemonic narrative of risky motherhood. In the dozens of blogs I reviewed, very few were written by women of color. The vast majority of them were written by white women, often in their late twenties to early forties. This face of motherhood in the blogosphere replicates the face of the idealized good mother: she is white, upper middle class, and heterosexual (and usually married). Importantly, it is not just the demographics of the blog writers that point to a postfeminist logic at work. What is equally significant is how the narrative of risky motherhood functions to sustain the underlying patriarchal power dynamics of good motherhood—that is, supporting a sense of women's appropriate role in the home—through a promotion of a child-first sensibility, even while the narrative frames the child-centered perspective through a discourse of choice and empowerment. Whether she is a stay-at-home mom or a working mother, the woman's emotional and intellectual focus is her children.

Catherine Connors, the author of the blog Her Bad Mother, is perhaps the best example of a postfeminist risky mother in the blogging world. Her descriptions of mothering are fraught with the type of engagement with risk that the mythical good mother would not encounter (or at least not discuss). She confesses in her bad mother manifesto: "I let them have cookies for breakfast. I let them stay up too late. . . . I have left my children alone in the bathtub. I have spanked my daughter."[54] Each of these statements indicates potentially risky behavior as defined by cultural guides on parenting: cookies at breakfast could lead to poor nutritional choices in the future, alone time in the bath could lead to drowning. Indeed, the active engagement of risk in this narrative is part of a larger postfeminist discourse that frames mothering as a series of empowered choices.[55] What makes the risky mother a feasible subjectivity in our contemporary social context with its focus on protecting children are two characteristics: first, her constant reaffirmation and centralization of her love for her children, and second, the limits to the risks the risky mother chooses to engage.[56] Catherine Connors ends a list of ten things she hates about motherhood (ranging from potty training to the tediousness of children's television shows) with a passionate declaration of love for her children: "Who make me grateful for my soft belly and squishy boobs and for my messy hair and my undereye circles and my scars . . . these miracles, my children, without whom I would not know love as completely as I do."[57] Risky mothers may voice temporary discontents, but such statements are always followed with a declaration about love and the wonderfulness of motherhood. The lists of complaints do very little to disrupt the underlying assumptions that guide the myth of the good mother: women are first and foremost mothers and mothering is fulfilling and natural. As with other examples of postfeminist discourse, the narrative of risky motherhood perpetuates roles and expectations for women that are quite traditional.

Like Catherine Connors, the risky mothers featured in the postfeminist narrative of risky motherhood raise happy, healthy, and ultimately safe children. The risks these mothers choose to take are small enough, although they are not always praised in public discourse. (For example, Connors's admission that she chose to stop breastfeeding because she did not like it opens her to critiques from breastfeeding advocates.) Connors offers common sense about weighing risks and benefits: "All that we have, then, is this: the measure of our hearts and the measure of our eyes and our ears and our good sense. Do we love our children as best we can? Do we keep them, as best we can, healthy in mind and body? Do we make sure that they laugh? Do they smile in our presence? That is enough. That must be enough."[58] The question that haunts her statement is exactly what is not enough. The second defining issue of the identity of the risky mother is the limit to the risks she takes. In the next section, I describe how postpartum depression is configured as an acceptable—even a normalized—risk.

The Risky Mother and Postpartum Disorders

The risky mother is an identity for all postfeminist mothers, not just those who suffer from a postpartum disorder. The characteristics of the risky mother— the fallible mother who (as socially expected) loves her children, the mother who chooses to engage in risky behavior—have important implications for our understanding of postpartum disorders. I argue that through the figure of the risky mother, postpartum depression is normalized. Although the normalization of postpartum depression partially destigmatizes postpartum depression (a goal of many postpartum self-help advocates), it rests on two strategies of reassurance, both of which undermine women's potential self-determination.

Normalizing Depression

When I claim that postpartum depression is normalized through the figure of the risky mother, I am pointing to the way postpartum depression is framed as a commonsense part of risky motherhood. Mary Douglas Vavrus explains that commonsense ideas are "beliefs that are historically determined yet so seemingly fundamental that they come to seem almost instinctive."[59] Postpartum depression becomes common sense not only because of its frequency (medical estimates suggests that it affects from 10 to 20 percent of new mothers), but also because in the postfeminist narrative of motherhood it is a natural part of being a risky mother. The normalization of postpartum depression occurs largely through two narrative strategies: medicalization and the destigmatization of symptoms.

Postpartum Depression and the Symptoms of Risky Mothering

In a review of Shields's memoir, Jane Brody of the *New York Times* offers this list of symptoms of postpartum depression: "[New mothers] may feel sad, hopeless, overwhelmed, unable to cope, irritable and afraid of harming themselves, their partners or their babies. Crying, uncontrollable mood swings, a fear of being alone, a lack of interest in the baby, loss of energy and motivation, withdrawal or isolation from friends and family, and an inability to make decisions or think clearly are also common symptoms."[60] Brody's list is echoed by most medical experts, and Shields, Armstrong, and the many other women who have given voice to the feelings of postpartum depression describe these symptoms frankly. Indeed, having these symptoms and recognizing them as symptoms of postpartum depression is framed as an important step toward recovery for women with postpartum depression.

Brooke Shields documents her descent into postpartum depression carefully and describes her feelings of hopelessness in detail. Comparing her experience to PMS, she explains, "In contrast, this felt like my life was over and I would never be happy again. I felt like a failure, and had tremendous guilt about not feeling close to my baby, but there was no way to explain the situation to anyone."[61] Looking back, Shields acknowledges a desperate wish for a "natural and healthy connection" with her daughter, but instead she felt "profound detachment."[62] Her detachment, her sadness, and her inability to sleep are represented in medical literature as the classic symptoms of postpartum depression. Similarly, Armstrong describes feelings of overwhelming sadness and, in her case, frustration and anxiety: "I'd get up in the morning having slept only an hour or two and couldn't imagine living another minute. The expanse of the day unfolded before me and I couldn't comprehend how I was going to distract my cranky baby for the next twelve hours."[63] Armstrong and Shields eventually sought help, but not until many weeks had gone by. Armstrong was familiar with depression (she had stopped taking her antidepressant before becoming pregnant), and when her daughter Leta was six weeks old she finally acknowledged that her ability to cope was deteriorating: "My daily life felt like torture. I struggled to make it from hour to hour. . . . I was trying to find the humor in all of it, but I couldn't ignore the crushing misery any longer."[64] She continued, "I was throwing up my hands. I couldn't do this unmedicated, and it was a decision I didn't make lightly."[65] Medication is also what Shields turned to, and she finally agreed (with her doctor's assistance) to try a low dose of Paxil.

Shields's and Armstrong's descriptions of their symptoms are nuanced and unflinching accounts of what it feels like to be depressed. However, although each account of postpartum depression in public discourse is unique, the emotions described by Shields and Armstrong are represented as experienced by most risky mothers. Women who participate in the narrative of risky motherhood who are not depressed describe their daily lives with their children with the same language—anxiety and depression, detachment and fear, anger and guilt, shame and loathing—that Shields and Armstrong use. I am not suggesting that all women have what might be diagnosed as postpartum depression but rather that the symptoms of postpartum depression (the negative emotions, the exhaustion, and so forth) that were once used only to describe women with postpartum depression are now represented as a normal part of mothering in the narrative of risky motherhood. Consider, for example, blogger and author Stefanie Wilder-Taylor's discussion of her anxiety regarding her daughter's health: "When Sadie has a few good days I relax only slightly, fully expecting the bad days to soon follow. . . . She is a beautiful baby and don't get me wrong, I appreciate her, but my antennae [are] always up and scanning—Is she eating less today? Why doesn't she want to wake up this morning? Why is she pale? Why can't she do algebra yet? Then I think, am I being paranoid? Is this anxiety making me imagine things that others aren't seeing? Or do the doctors worry too but not want to worry me?"[66] One can read in Wilder-Taylor's description of her concerns a sense of the persistent worries and anxiety that are simply part of life for the risky mother.

Katie, a mommy blogger, also uses the language of postpartum depression when she describes her feelings. She offers this description of her daughter: "*She still wont crawl.* I know. Its not the worst thing in the world. But to me it is! I mean, she is 10.5 months old for crying out loud and she just sits there! When I take her to playdates with other babies her age, they crawl and pull up and even walk . . . but not Ellie Kate. She sits. And I feel dumb. I feel like a failure. I feel embar[r]assed."[67] These feelings of embarrassment and failure are echoed by mothers who explicitly identify as having postpartum depression. Kimberly, a mother who blogs about her experiences with postpartum depression, recalls her feelings when she was told she would have to stop breastfeeding: "I remember crying as the ER doctor wrote out PREDNISONE on the script pad. 'This will pass through your breast milk, so you'll need to switch to formula.' I was giving in. In a sense I almost started to grieve because I knew that giving up breastfeeding would ultimately mean giving up the only bond that I had with my son. 'You're a weak person. How could I put my needs before my baby's? I am a horrible Mom.'"[68] In sum, many of physical symptoms and emotions women with postpartum depression experience are no longer relegated to the realm of postpartum depression. Although varying in seriousness (the paralyzing anxiety of Armstrong compared to Katie's feelings of failure), the symptoms of postpartum depression are represented as symptoms of risky motherhood. The fact that both mothers who have experienced postpartum depression and those who have not write so openly about the feelings and experiences after childbirth makes it clear that they are almost universal. Such openness is a significant step in the process of destigmatizing the experience of postpartum depression. Women with postpartum depression who are feeling sad, angry, guilty, and anxious are often in emotional turmoil in part because the emotions they are experiencing are not accepted (or expected) in the myth of good motherhood. However, within the postfeminist narrative of risky motherhood, such emotions are expected, and they are discussed openly and often with humor.

Medicalization and the Risky Mother

The lesson we learn in public discourse about motherhood is that it is tough: mothering is full of ups and downs, and no mother is ever perfect. Because no mother is ever perfect, all mothers in this discourse are always risky mothers. Risky mothers are risky because they are human, and they have human flaws. Some mothers are addicts, and sometimes they need to slip away for a cigarette or a drink.[69] Some mothers do not care about cooking, and they feed their children prepared food. Some mothers have a physiological propensity toward depression and/or anxiety, and without medical help they are irritable with and detached from their children. Consider this explanation from the blogger at Postpartum Progress: "Being a parent is tough business, and for those of us with perinatal mood and anxiety disorders I'd venture to say it's even tougher. We start off on the wrong foot from the very start. This leads to even more self-doubt, even more guilt, and even more second-guessing."[70] Risky mothers with postpartum depression are not unlike the mothers who do not experience postpartum depression. They are just like them, with one small difference, here described as starting off on the wrong foot. As constructed in public discourse, this last mother—a risky mother like the rest—is unique in that her riskiness is embodied and can be easily treated. In this section, I focus on the risky mother with postpartum depression and examine how postpartum depression is medicalized in public discourse and how that medicalization contributes to the normalization of the disorder.

The link between medicalization and destigmatization has long been recognized by postpartum self-help advocates who worked for a medical diagnosis even while attempting to maintain the understanding of postpartum disorders as contextualized in the experience of and expectations of mothering. Shields explains the relief a woman can feel when she receives a diagnosis: "In a strange way, it was comforting to me when my obstetrician told me that my feelings of extreme despair and my suicidal thoughts were directly tied to a biochemical shift in my body. Once we admit that postpartum depression is a serious medical condition, then the treatment becomes more available and socially acceptable."[71] The dominance of the psychiatric molecular gaze is clear in the news coverage of postpartum depression and in both of the memoirs I analyze. Definitions of postpartum depression, such as the one Shields offers above, routinely rely on biological explanations of depression. Reporter Susan Gilbert offers this explanation: "Doctors have long thought that postpartum depression is related at least in part to the sharp decline in estrogen that occurs immediately after childbirth. . . . Precisely how a drop in estrogen might set off depression is unknown, but studies show a relationship between the hormone and several neurotransmitters that influence mood."[72]

An official diagnosis removes much of the stigma of postpartum depression. As Shields and many other writers explain, depression is a real disease, and it is characterized as one women have no real control over. Responsibility for a disease is directly related to both blame and the potential for stigma, as is the case with a smoker who has lung cancer or (as I discuss in the next chapter) a sexually active woman with HPV. The careful construction of postpartum depression as physiological—a problem of neurotransmitters and hormones— allows risky mothers to diminish both the blame and the stigma associated with not loving their children as society expects them to. This may be part of the reason why actor Tom Cruise incurred such a backlash when he asserted in 2005 that postpartum depression could be controlled through exercise and vitamins. In a *New York Times* editorial, Shields harshly critiques Cruise and in response to his "ridiculous rant" suggests that "comments like those made by Tom Cruise are a disservice to mothers everywhere. To suggest that I was wrong to take drugs to deal with my depression, and that instead I should have taken vitamins and exercised shows an utter lack of understanding about postpartum depression and childbirth in general."[73] Shields's explanation of the disease in her editorial removes all of her agency and thus her ability to exert control or receive blame: "Postpartum depression is caused by the hormonal shifts that occur after childbirth. . . . This change in hormone levels can lead to reactions that range from restlessness to irritability to feelings of sadness and hopelessness."[74] Katherine Stone, the blogger at Postpartum Progress is also explicit about women's blamelessness: "You are not defective, or weak, or a bad person. . . . What we do know is that this is not your fault. Don't beat yourself up for getting a common and treatable illness."[75]

As with the women who test positive for the BRCA1 or BRCA2 gene mutations, risky mothers find themselves facing an embodied risk (a gene mutation, a neurotransmitter/hormone malfunction) that they did not choose. Their responsibility hinges not on the appearance of the mutation or depression but rather on the actions they are expected to take as the necessary next step. For women with postpartum disorders, that next step is treatment (usually through psychiatric pharmaceuticals). Much like Shields, Armstrong relies on a biochemical explanation for her postpartum depression. For both women, psychiatric drugs are a pivotal part of the treatment plan. For Armstrong, resuming her course of antidepressants after childbirth is significant because it confirms two aspects of the medicalized definition of postpartum depression. First, Armstrong embodies one of the strongest predictors of postpartum depression noted in psychiatric research: she has previously experienced depression. Second, her treatment plan confirms that depression is chemical in nature and is thus easily treatable. As reporter Jane Brody explains, postpartum depression is most often treated with SSRIs (selective serotonin reuptake inhibitors), a popular class of antidepressants. Armstrong reflects on her experience, "But I finally gave in and realized I couldn't climb out of the hole by myself, and I had come to accept that I would never be off medication. . . . Sometimes I had bad days, sometimes bad weeks, but the medication enabled me to cope, to see a way out and over those times. I was not ashamed of any of this."[76] In fact, she jokes frequently throughout the book about her need to "pop a pill once a day to connect certain chemicals in my brain."[77]

One of the problems with the medicalization of postpartum depression is the lack of attention paid to the social context of the disorder. Davi Johnson notes the tendency of psychiatric language to individualize subjects; in the case of postpartum depression, risky mothers are represented as having a particular biochemical makeup that can be differentiated through a variety of diagnostic techniques.[78] The medicalization of postpartum disorders thus offers women few options other than medical pharmaceuticals for recovery. I discuss the problem of decontextualization—and a (perhaps) surprising solution—at the end of the chapter. For now, I want to suggest that not only does medicalization do significant work in terms of destigmatizing postpartum depression, but it also normalizes it—literally by making it seem natural, an occurrence that can be expected, even if it does not happen to every woman. Shields illustrates this point as she perseveres in finding women who are willing to talk about their experiences with postpartum depression: "Soon, because of how honest I was about my terrifying experience, people started saying things like 'Oh, no, I had it real bad.' Or 'Believe me, I know, my aunt was hospitalized.' One person told me, 'It got so bad, a friend of mine was actually standing on the window ledge of their apartment while her baby was in the next room.'"[79] The more she talked, the more women she found who shared a stream of experiences that were similar to hers. The statistics that are frequently offered for postpartum depression in public discourse suggest that as many as one-fifth of all new mothers suffer from postpartum depression; the disease is no longer extraordinary. The pervasive sense in public discourse that postpartum depression is common is due in part to narratives such as those offered by Shields and Armstrong, reports that numerous other celebrities have suffered from postpartum depression, and the overall culture of motherhood in which risky mothers give voice to their despair, not just to their joy and happiness.[80] The result is declarations such as this, from *Time* magazine: "Postpartum depression is a familiar rite of new parenthood. Feelings of emptiness, sadness, and anxiety settle in after the birth of a child, and in severe cases last for months."[81] It is possible at this point that postpartum depression may be traveling the same path as breast cancer, which Barbara Ehrenreich suggests has become a "rite of passage" for middle-aged American women.[82]

Depressed Risky Mothers and the Risk of Harm

The normalization of postpartum depression through medicalization and the universalization of symptoms by risky mothers in blogs, memoirs, and news reports—including mothers who have not been diagnosed with postpartum depression—prompts several questions. How does one know if one has postpartum depression if many (if not most) new mothers experience the emotions (anxiety, anger, sadness) that are identified as symptoms of postpartum depression? Do risky mothers with postpartum depression pose a different risk to their children than mothers who are not officially diagnosed with postpartum depression? Risky mothers who identify as having postpartum depression are represented in mainstream discourse as more concerned with two issues—thoughts of hurting themselves and thoughts of hurting their children—than the risky mothers who do not describe themselves as having postpartum depression. I noted earlier that the narrative of risky motherhood creates space for mothers to take small risks with their children that are deemed largely inconsequential. One of the primary reasons these risks can be engaged is the larger discourse of love for children and the very child-centered nature of risky motherhood. For the risky mothers with postpartum depression, the risk of harm to a child and to oneself is present, and it is represented as more serious than, for example, the risk of leaving a child alone to spend a few quiet minutes in the bathroom. However, as serious as the risks posed by the depressed risky mother are, they are also consistently diminished and incorporated into the larger and accepted discourse of risky motherhood through two strategies of reassurance that relate directly to the status of the risky mother as a vulnerable empowered woman: an emphasis on surveillance and the construction of a monstrous mother figure. Both of these strategies are suspect from a feminist perspective on women's health because they ultimately place all women under the surveillance of medical practitioners, friends, and family members and because they condemn women who do not fit the risky mother model.

The Risky Mother and Empowerment through Surveillance

As an iteration of the vulnerable empowered woman, the risky mother's vulnerabilities are all too clear. Her vulnerabilities are human fallibilities; she may make human errors and choices that may place her child at risk. A depressed risky mother is also represented in mainstream discourse as having an additional biological vulnerability to depression. Recognizing this vulnerability is the key to the empowerment of the risky mother, for once it is recognized, she can seek treatment. In this section, I discuss how surveillance—by oneself and by others—is transformed into a mechanism of empowerment for the risky mother.

Neoliberal subjects are encouraged to engage in self-discipline. The focus on the self shifts the focus from the problem of postpartum depression (in this case) as a collective, systemic problem to a problem of many individuals.[83] Davi Johnson explains, "The contemporary formation of 'madness' facilitates the spread of biopower [power over bodies] by rendering virtually all aspects of daily life as focal points for self-observation, self-regulation, and self-improvement."[84] As a method of empowerment, surveillance of the self through what Foucault describes as the clinical gaze also prompts women's further engagement with biomedicine. Specifically, risky mothers are asked to become diagnosticians—to recognize certain emotions as evidence of postpartum depression and seek treatment before they do harm.

After giving birth, women are encouraged to engage in self-surveillance by other risky mothers and by their doctors, families, and friends. For example, at the end of her memoir, Brooke Shields gives instructions to new mothers: "If you think you might be suffering from any kind of postpartum mood disorder, or are aware of some preexisting condition in your life that could lead to it, DO NOT WASTE TIME! Get help right away. Even if you don't have a history of depression or haven't experienced any of the aforementioned precipitating events, but what you are feeling seems out of reach beyond those few days of symptoms associated with the baby blues, then consult a professional."[85] Much of what Shields is asking for in this quotation depends on the mother's interpretation of her thoughts and feelings. Shields prompts one interpretation (if what you are feeling seems "out of reach") that aligns with the understanding of postpartum depression as worse than simple baby blues or the usual frustrations that come with mothering. Shields is engaging in the language of self-diagnosis and asking other mothers to do the same.

Americans are astute in analyzing their emotional states, and they are willing to understand emotional experiences that fall outside the prescribed norm as indicating a "medical problem" that needs treatment.[86] The sense that individuals pick up on psychiatric language to describe their everyday experiences is relevant to my understanding of public discourse about postpartum depression and risky motherhood.[87] Such is certainly the case for risky mothers (including those who may not qualify in the ambiguous world of psychiatric practice for an actual diagnosis of postpartum depression). Gwyneth Paltrow provides an example of this as she picks up on the framework of postpartum depression to describe her experiences after the birth of her son: "You know,

I had postnatal depression after [my second child] Moses. I didn't know I had it until after it was over. I just didn't know what was wrong with me. . . . I felt really out of my body. I felt really disconnected. I felt really down; I felt pessimistic."[88] Paltrow's description suggests that she is well aware of the diagnosis of postpartum depression and, looking back, can use that language and a psychiatric framework to understand her emotional states. The language of postpartum depression serves to validate; it "constitutes a 'truth'" that is closely connected with medical authority.[89]

Like Paltrow, other mothers with postpartum depression spend time not only recording but also analyzing their emotions. Because Heather Armstrong was treated for depression before her first pregnancy, she was aware that it was possible that she might experience postpartum depression. She relates, "Before Leta was born Jon and I talked at length about what we would do if I slipped into a postpartum funk, but for some reason I didn't think it would ever happen, especially since I had made it through those first crucial months. But the funk finally happened, and it wasn't so much a simple slipping into as it was a full-fledged belly flop."[90] As she records in her memoir, she was paying careful attention to her emotional state after Leta was born and she was using a variety of strategies—getting out of the house, watching television—to cope with her anxiety. She explains, "For several weeks I felt like I was fighting a losing battle. I was doing everything I knew how to do to cope with feelings of hopelessness and frustration and an overwhelming sense of failure."[91] Her coping strategies did not work, and what is significant about Armstrong's postpartum depression narrative is that she performed self-surveillance perfectly: she knew her strategies were not working. She knew that her emotional state had become, in her words, "life-threatening," and because of this knowledge she could take steps to mitigate the risks she posed to herself and her daughter.[92] Yet even though Armstrong took steps to help herself—doing exactly what Shields instructs women to do—she did not get better. Her description of the decision to finally check into a psychiatric ward is remarkable because of the level of her self-knowledge about her emotional state:

> My anxiety had only gotten worse since I started seeing a therapist three months earlier. It was so bad that it choked me every day, and sometimes I couldn't even walk because my body was paralyzed with anxiety. I'd tried over ten different medications and each one had made my anxiety worse. The depression came and went and then came again, but the anxiety was constant. I could barely eat anything and couldn't sleep, even though I'd tried every sleeping pill available at the pharmacy. I

wanted to commit suicide if only because then I wouldn't have to feel the pain of being awake anymore. I couldn't believe that I didn't feel better. I couldn't believe that it had been three months and I DIDN'T FEEL ANY BETTER.[93]

Armstrong tracked her physical symptoms (paralysis, inability to eat and sleep) along with her deteriorating emotional state. Her decision to go to the hospital was made with a tinge of desperation and the hope that the hospital stay would work where the other treatments had not.

Armstrong is not unique in her ability to track her emotional thoughts, recognize the severity of her symptoms, engage in self-help/coping, and seek treatment. Because in the larger narrative of risky motherhood mothers engage in public discussions of their fallibilities and bad mommy moments, risky mothers engage in public analysis of their private emotional states. Self-surveillance—even self-regulation of emotion—becomes not a private but a public function of the risky mother. Consider, for example, a blogger who self-identifies as having postpartum depression. She begins a post in November 2009 with this statement: "I must digress from my journey into madness a little bit as it seems to be stirring up some pretty icky emotions and I don't like icky emotions. Icky emotions lead to bad thoughts, bad thoughts lead to anxiety, anxiety leads to meltdowns, meltdowns lead to locking myself in the bathroom, and meltdowns lead to an overall shitty day and I don't like shitty days."[94] The blogger recognizes the spiraling pattern of emotions.

As a method of empowerment, self-surveillance as a form of self-discipline promises risky mothers suffering from postpartum depression a path to better mental health, thus enabling them to avoid the more serious risks they pose to themselves and their children. One guest blogger from Postpartum Progress describes her own recovery as empowerment through understanding her emotions: "over the last two years i've definitely learned some tricks. i know how to sit with my anxiety better. how not to let it snowball."[95] With empowerment through self-surveillance and discipline, this blogger better understands herself (she knows what anxiety feels like and she knows what to do when she feels anxiety), she can control or discipline her own emotional states, and, most importantly, with this knowledge she can continue her job as a mother. With the power that self-knowledge brings, risky mothers are enabled to continue down the often rocky path of motherhood, at times (for depressed mothers) with some medical assistance. The public nature of self-surveillance on the part of risky mothers functions in discourse as a form of reassurance that the risks depressed risky mothers take are always being managed by the mothers themselves. However, such management is supplemented in public discourse by surveillance of mothers by others. This form of surveillance is also presented as a form of empowerment, although (like self-surveillance), I would suggest that it operates as a form of regulatory discipline.

In case a woman's own ability to interpret and report her emotional state is not adequate, surveillance by others ensures that a depressed mother will receive treatment. As presented in public discourse, surveillance by others—parents, friends, spouses, doctors, and even the state—helps the risky mother recognize that her emotions are "out of reach." Again, postpartum depression is not represented in this discourse as a bad or stigmatized disease; it is common enough that women deserve the empowerment that comes with the help of surveillance by others. Consider, for example, this discussion of a New Jersey screening law in the *New York Times*: "'They don't think they're entitled to be depressed,' Dr. Stotland says. 'People tell you that it's the happiest time of your life and you're mortified if you don't feel like that.' So it's good news that the State Senate and the Assembly have unanimously passed a bill requiring New Jersey doctors and other health professionals to screen new mothers for symptoms of postpartum depression. It also requires childbirth facilities to give their patients (including fathers) information about this illness."[96] The reporter follows Dr. Stotland's statement with praise for the New Jersey law. Stotland's understanding of mothers as not feeling entitled to be depressed is important. While the normalization of postpartum depression in the narrative of risky motherhood suggests that women are entitled to be depressed, women who do not yet feel this entitlement (a risky mother who is not yet able to engage in self-surveillance and the disciplining of emotional states through psychiatric treatment) need assistance in the form of surveillance and outreach by others. The system of surveillance around the depressed mother emphasizes her vulnerability at the same time that it promises her empowerment. Furthermore, such a system suggests that all risky mothers—all mothers in the postfeminist narrative of risky motherhood—are potentially vulnerable to postpartum depression and should thus be surveilled. Although postpartum depression is normalized in this discourse, voices in the postpartum depression narrative agree that it must be treated because it is a disease.

Brooke Shields's memoir offers extensive examples of empowerment through surveillance by others. She recalls, for example, traveling from New York to Los Angeles soon after the birth of her daughter and running into acquaintances on the plane, one of whom was a doctor. Shields describes their encounter: "He kept looking at me with a warm yet inquisitive expression. He asked me a few times how I was, and I remember thinking, Did someone put a sign on my forehead that says, *Not doing well?* I said, 'Fine,' but each time he pressed on like a heat-seeking missile. Suddenly he volunteered the information that his wife had had a hard time after their first child was born."[97] Although this doctor had no knowledge of Shields's emotional turbulence (or that she had begun taking Paxil), he was performing surveillance of a risky mother. Because all new mothers are potentially vulnerable to postpartum depression, he was searching for the signs and symptoms. Even more remarkable, near the end of his conversation with her, he gave her information about postpartum mood disorders and quickly switched seats with his wife so that she could share her experience with Shields. Shields remembers listening to his wife describe her experiences, and notes that "I kept hearing some of her words in my head, like 'self doubt' and 'panic.' I started thinking it was possible that I, too, was going through something serious."[98] This example is not an abrupt mental health intervention; Shields does not find herself incarcerated in a mental hospital. However, it does exactly what I suggest is the function of surveillance of risky mothers by others: her acquaintances' surveillance prompts her own self-surveillance and her own recognition that something was not right. Shields presents this surveillance as empowering her to recognize and then seek treatment for her own emotions.

Once she was under a physician's care, Shields made good progress in overcoming her depression. However, she continued to engage in self-surveillance of her emotions, worried that she would relapse again: "I did have some nightmares about the black cloud descending again. I was far from fully recovered, and sometimes I dreamed that I had lost my daughter or that, no matter how hard I tried, I couldn't complete a task that involved her care."[99] Shields paid careful attention to these feelings, talking at length with her therapist about what were "common parental worries" and what might be another sign of postpartum depression. Her therapist's explanation largely confirmed the continuum of nondepressed and depressed risky mothers: "Any number of normal maternal issues could be causing the fears or the dreams, but as long as they didn't escalate further or start to strongly interfere with my day, then I was probably experiencing the general angst that comes with being a mom."[100] Interestingly, it is precisely because of this continuum—of angst versus escalated angst—that Shields and all risky mothers need to be under constant surveillance. Outside of the realm of medicine—where doctors and nurses offer screening and even friendly medical acquaintances watch with inquisitive eyes—other members of the risky mother's social circle take up the job of surveillance. Shields is quite aware of this, noting that it changes the dynamic between her and her husband: "Sometimes he'd wait and watch my reactions to Rowan's crying or to any of the daily frustrations I had. It was as if he wanted to make sure none of it would put me over the edge, like it might have in the recent past. He would quietly sigh in relief when I didn't become upset."[101]

Much like the risky mother is prompted to analyze her emotions and recognize those that are out of bounds, her friends and family do the same, and they do it using much of the same medical parlance. In other words, all of the people involved engage in a clinical gaze to understand the mother's behavior. The Postpartum Progress blog encourages this surveillance as a means of helping the new mother. Writing to new fathers, Katherine Stone explains, "Perhaps you can't exactly put your finger on it, but you know she's not acting like you thought she would. Maybe she seems sad all the time and can't stop crying. Maybe she keeps saying she's not a good mom even though you tell her over and over again that she's doing just fine. Maybe she's really angry with you all the time now, or she's worrying nonstop and can't relax."[102] Stone hopes that when her behavior seems "abnormal" (although common), friends and family will push her to recognize it as such and seek medical help. To assist in this process, Stone tells new fathers to learn the symptoms. Thus, fathers—and family and friends—are asked to distinguish between healthy and unhealthy behaviors, between angst and escalated angst. They are concerned diagnosticians, watching the risky mother and prompting treatment when necessary.

Once she is empowered with knowledge—whether it is given to her by others or she finds it on her own—and a correct interpretation of her emotional experiences, the depressed risky mother is well on her way to recovery. The discourse of surveillance in the postpartum narrative holds the promise that the depressed woman is still a risky mother, the contemporary, postfeminist iteration of the good mother. Importantly, the potential for bad mothering does not disappear in the narrative of risky motherhood. In the myth of good motherhood, the dichotomous figures of the good mother and the bad mother work together to construct good mothering: the perfection of the good mother depends in part on the imperfection of bad mothering. In the postfeminist narrative of risky motherhood, the same good/bad dichotomy exists: the bad mother figure plays an important role in constructing the meaning of good mothering. For clarity, I discuss the postfeminist iteration of the good mother/bad mother dichotomy using the terms "risky mother" and "monstrous mother." In the narrative of postfeminist risky motherhood, the monstrous mother normalizes the risks of the depressed risky mother by demarcating what risks can and cannot be tolerated. And that dividing line is determined through the diagnosis of postpartum psychosis.

The Risky Mother and the Monstrous Mother

In the postfeminist discourse of motherhood, all risky mothers are represented as existing on a continuum. All engage in risky mothering, but there is a qualitative difference in the types of risks engaged. In part, this construction of a continuum echoes the understanding of postpartum disorders in medical discourse, which presents postpartum disorders on a continuum of "baby blues," postpartum depression, and postpartum psychosis. I have concentrated in my analysis thus far on the representations of the depressed risky mother: the mother who has a diagnosis (whether provided by herself or by a doctor) of postpartum depression.[103] However, women with postpartum psychosis do not easily fit within the risky mother framework. In public discourse, the mother with postpartum psychosis—particularly one who acts in her psychotic state—is characterized as fundamentally different from risky mothers. This demarcation is a strategy of reassurance; it suggests that only psychotic mothers fail to mitigate the risks of mental illness.

Women who actually harm their children haunt the narratives of depressed risky mothers. Shields explains her own early resistance to the label of postpartum depression: "Postpartum depression was a crazy person's affliction, and I associated it only with those people who harmed their kids by doing things like driving the car into a lake. I was certainly not in that category. I had no intention of ever harming my baby."[104] Shields's oblique reference to Susan Smith, a woman who killed her children by strapping them into their car seats and pushing her car into a lake, characterizes Smith as distinctly different than herself. Shields's perspective on her disease delineates the difference: "And I had to admit to being a legitimate member of the depressed mommy society. Did this mean that I was crazy or that I was destined to be on the six o'clock news because of my inevitable actions? Of course not."[105] Depressed mommies, to use her phrase, are not "crazy mommies." Crazy mommies are monstrous in this narrative; they are mothers who "fail in their parental roles so grievously as to cause serious harm or even death to their children or others."[106]

The line between "depression" and "psychosis" is ambiguous in medical literature, but in public discourse depressed risky mothers go to great lengths to distinguish psychosis—and the monstrous acts caused by psychosis—from depression. In 2009, for example, postpartum activists were in an uproar over an episode of *Private Practice*, a medical TV drama, that featured a plotline about postpartum depression. The show's staff had consulted postpartum depression experts and Postpartum Support International had crafted the language for a public service announcement to air during a commercial break. However, the show's plot was clearly about postpartum psychosis, not postpartum depression; it centered on a mother who was considering drowning her child in the bathtub. Katherine Stone of Postpartum Progress expressed her outrage, noting that the show only offered a portrayal of "some out-of-control woman committing or attempting to commit infanticide" instead of giving information about the commonness and treatability of postpartum depression.[107] Further, the show suggested implicitly that a mother with postpartum psychosis always "ends up killing their child."

Stone is careful to note that women with postpartum psychosis do not always kill their children, and indeed, the monstrous mother is depicted as a woman who follows through on her thoughts. Not surprisingly, Andrea Yates is often used as a touchstone for the monstrous mother construct (Yates is implicitly referenced in the *Private Practice* episode). Although much work has been done in public discourse to rehabilitate Yates's image—usually by referring to a medicalized understanding of the postpartum period and explaining the medical "facts" behind postpartum psychosis—in the voices of depressed risky mothers, she is represented as standing for exactly what they are not.[108] In postpartum depression narratives, descriptions of thoughts of harm on the part of depressed risky mothers are immediately followed by a reassurance that the mother knows that she would never actually be able to harm her children. Brooke Shields describes her own horror at her thoughts: "During what was becoming one of the darkest points in my life, I sat holding my newborn and could not avoid the image of her flying through the air and hitting the wall in front of me. I was horrified, and although I knew deep in my soul that I would not harm her, the image all but destroyed me."[109] Shields does not deny the seriousness of her thoughts, but she follows them with the assurance that she would not actually harm her daughter.

Lauren Hale's description on her blog of her decision to enter a mental hospital also invokes Yates as the monstrous mother and points to the exact line between a risky and monstrous mothers: the act of harm. In four blog entries, Hale relates her breakdown, beginning with the birth of her special-needs daughter. At her lowest, right before entering the hospital, Hale thought about harming her children: "My thin strand of reality shredding, I turned to the voices. They started to push me toward the brink of the canyon. I didn't have much fight left inside. Home alone, it would be so easy. The monsters were gaining ground. Their battering ram tediously close to knocking down the last door I had shored up against them, I went to our bedroom and closed the door, disgusted with myself."[110] Sinking into her bed, she calls her husband, and then her doctor. She explains that she needs help and heads to the emergency room. There, she tells her a nurse her horrible thoughts, "horrible things like not bonding with my child and wanting to smother her with a pillow." As she speaks with an emergency room doctor, she finally offers this plea: "I'm here because I do not want to be Andrea Yates. I don't want to be Andrea Yates. Please, keep me from being Andrea Yates."[111] Lauren Hale's narrative suggests that although risky mothers can have thoughts of harming their children, they absolutely cannot act on them. Treatment can return the mothers on the verge of becoming monstrous back to living as risky mothers. In the narratives, the fact that risky mothers do not cross the line is a testament to the success of surveillance by self and others and the miracle of medical treatment.

The resurrection of the good/bad mother dichotomy works to normalize the risk of the average depressed (or even psychotic) risky mother. As Shields suggests, she is not going to appear on the six o'clock news. However, in the process of normalizing postpartum depression, the narrative of risky motherhood has re-created a dichotomy that reinforces the essential badness of mothers who harm their children. The coverage of the second Yates verdict in 2006 hints at her status as a monstrous mother, for although she was found not guilty by reason of insanity (suggesting that the jury accepted the argument that while she was in a psychotic state, she did not know right from wrong and had no control over her actions) the coverage continued to reinforce Yates's monstrosity. One juror remarked, "Although she's treated, I think she's worse than she was before. I think she'll probably need treatment for the rest of her life."[112] Unlike the treatment given to women before they harm their children (or to women who are simply depressed and/or anxious), Yates's treatment will never return her to the role of a good, regular risky mother. Coverage of other incidents of infanticide demonstrates similar condemnation, even when mental illness is clearly identified in the coverage as a factor. In reaction to a case of child abandonment that led to the child's death, one citizen said, "It's mind-boggling that another human being could abandon an innocent newborn."[113] The graphic description of the baby's body and its death reaffirms the monstrosity of the mother: "In the case of Michael [the name given to the baby after it died], the child was born alive and possibly abandoned on the snow-covered Hempstead Golf and Country Club or dumped in a garbage can, and dragged to the middle of the street by an animal, police suspect. The boy's crushed, naked body was so disfigured that detectives were initially unable to determine its sex or race."[114] The father of one murdered child, whose mother was represented as suffering from psychosis, offered no recourse for redemption: "She was a sweet person and I still love her, but she needs to pay the ultimate price for what she has done."[115]

Mothers who harm their children because of psychosis are depicted as failing to enact the mode of empowerment that is offered to risky mothers: they do not recognize their own emotions as dangerous and they do not seek treatment. Their failure to seek treatment opens the doors to the type of judgment that the father discussed above offers regarding the mother of his child. Reports of Yates's long struggle with mental illness prompt attention to her inability to correctly interpret and seek treatment for her emotional states. A lengthy article in *Time*, for example, describes her mental illness as a "secret history" that she shared with no one until it was too late. For example, after the birth of her first child, Noah, she had a vision: "The image of a knife crossed her mind, flickering into a scene of somebody being stabbed."[116] Her next move was critical: "She dismissed it and never told Rusty, who says he learned of it only after her arrest."[117] In the Yates case, the media quickly distributed blame to a number of people. Yates is represented as failing to understand her own emotional state, but news reports during both the original trial and the second trial point to her husband's lack of attention and her doctor's misinterpretation of her symptoms. One article, for example, describes Rusty's inability to watch his wife properly in 1999: "Andrea seemed tired and preoccupied on the drive home to Texas, recalls Rusty, who assumed she was suffering from the aftereffects of the flu, which they all had had."[118] After she had a breakdown but seemed on the path to recovery, Rusty "admits that he asked nothing else," noting that he "didn't want to pry."[119] However, in the discourse of surveillance in the context of postpartum depression and the risky mother, the role of husbands, family members, and friends is to help empower the vulnerable woman to recognize her own need for medical assistance. Yates's brother reports, "She would not ask us for help. Maybe she didn't know how."[120] As a monstrous mother, Yates was only vulnerable, never empowered. Public discourse about Yates recognizes the depth of her psychosis (no discussion of her case fails to take into account her mental illness), but her actions are, in the language of a *Newsweek* article, "unspeakable."[121]

Implications of Surveillance and the Monstrous Mother

At the heart of the process of normalizing postpartum depression is the distinctly elite figure of the risky mother. In blogs, news coverage, and memoirs about postpartum depression, women are positioned within a framework of postfeminist privilege. Like the women of the prophylactic mastectomy narratives—and indeed of postfeminist women's health discourse more broadly—risky mothers share a narrow realm of experiences. In this section, I briefly discuss the problems with surveillance as empowerment and the re-creation of the good/bad divide through the subjectivities of the risky and monstrous mothers and then discuss how these two strategies of reassurance are even more problematic for the women who exist outside the idealized version of postfeminist motherhood.

Both surveillance as a mode of empowerment and the reinvigoration of a bad mother figure (the monstrous mother) put risky mothers in a perilous position that can be less than empowering. Surveillance by those with a clinical gaze relies upon a medical understanding of motherhood, and surveillance of new mothers by themselves, their friends, and family members extends the power of the clinical gaze into the familial/domestic sphere. Because all mothers are represented as potentially depressed, all are subjects of surveillance. All behaviors are potentially signs of "riskier" nurturing, and risky mothers are never quite free of the gaze of others—or of their own gaze. Shields, for example, recognizes one of the fundamental issues underlying conversations with her husband: trust. "Chris looked at me with a slightly worried expression and asked if I had gone off my medicine. I don't blame him for being concerned about my mental state, but I got very insulted. . . . Was I really that unstable? Trust seemed to be an issue, and I feared that the people close to me would never trust me to be whole or completely sane again."[122] Although Shields reaches the point by the end of the memoir where she does feel trusted—and trusts herself—I would suggest that the surveillance of all risky mothers does indeed signal a lack of trust. Mothers in the postfeminist narrative of risky motherhood all engage in risks. While most risks engaged are harmless, the potential for the risks to be more serious (supported by the presence in this discourse of the monstrous mother) supports the surveillance of all mothers.

This kind of surveillance echoes what Douglas and Michaels describe as the intense scrutiny of mothers and pregnant women in public spaces. The concerned citizen interrupting a pregnant woman ordering coffee to remind her that caffeine is harmful to her unborn child is offering the same sort of assistance as the concerned friend or spouse reflecting on his/her partner's emotional behavior. The young breastfeeding mother who monitors her food and alcohol intake is operating in much the same, self-disciplining way as the mother who carefully monitors her emotions. The end result of such surveillance is the disciplining of all mothers because of concern for the child. Risky mothers take risks, but their risk-taking behavior is monitored carefully by others. Although some voices in public discourse oppose methods of surveillance such as screening laws (like the New Jersey law) because of the medicalization of motherhood (for example, *Time* suggests that "increased screening could lead to an increase in mothers being prescribed psychiatric medications"), they are rare. In a response to the *Time* article pointing to the potential flaws of screening, postpartum bloggers and experts joined together to write a letter to the editor. They argued that "it is no more medicalizing motherhood to identify and treat PPD than it is to identify and treat gestational diabetes, which is universally screened for and occurs in only 3.5 percent of mothers."[123] The authors position surveillance through increased screening as a way to ensure that women receive appropriate treatment: "Many women will tell you that screening saved their lives, and others who were not screened wish they had been so they could have received treatment sooner." Surveillance by doctors is then directly linked to women's potential empowerment, as "a well trained and educated physician will know when to refer the patient on to a specialist who can inform her various treatment options and monitor her to ensure the treatment she chooses is effective."[124]

The responders to the *Time* article clearly demonstrate that medicalization (in this case, through medical surveillance) is often advocated by individuals who see a clear need for medical intervention. Nikolas Rose points to this very dynamic in his critique of medicalization as an explanatory mechanism in social analysis: "Medicalisation implies passivity on the part of the medicalized. . . . [but] [w]ith notable exceptions (children, prisoners, people deemed mentally ill and admitted to hospital under compulsion), doctors do not force diagnostic labels on resistant individuals."[125] My concern with the position taken by the advocates arguing for a medicalized version of postpartum depression is that when understood through a larger postfeminist narrative about motherhood, the process of medicalization centers the problem on the biological processes of individual women. The postfeminist narrative of risky motherhood—focusing on the self-disciplining, self-aware, and self-reflexive neoliberal subject—offers no resistance to the individualizing force of medicalization. Combined, a postfeminist narrative of motherhood plus the medicalizing of postpartum disorders emphasizes the risky mother's position as a vulnerable empowered subject, one who is responsible for the mitigation of risk. The emphasis on surveillance by self and others as the mechanism of empowerment for the risky mother captures the problems of medicalization within a postfeminist, neoliberal narrative. Simply put, when a woman fails to receive treatment, the discourse of surveillance positions responsibility for that failure squarely on her shoulders. As Shields explains, "There were no medals handed out to people who chose to stay miserable. Medicine existed for a reason. Not treating the illness would be irresponsible."[126]

Because the normalizing of postpartum depression includes a bad mother figure, the risky mother who fails to receive treatment is quickly condemned. Through the construction of a monstrous mother figure—a mother with psychosis who acts on her "abnormal" thoughts—the depiction of postpartum depression in the narrative of real motherhood continues the stigmatization of postpartum disorders, if only for one segment of the population. I am certainly not arguing that harming children in any way is acceptable; what I am suggesting is that in separating psychosis from depression, risky mothers engage in the very process of stigmatization that they are dedicated to fighting against. By basing the social acceptance of postpartum depression on the stigmatization of women with postpartum psychosis, risky mothers are potentially undermining their status as good mothers. One way that risky mothers with postpartum depression are realigned with the myth of good motherhood is through the medicalization of postpartum depression. Postpartum psychosis is also treated as a biomedical phenomenon. The salient difference, then, between the risky mother and the monstrous mother in public discourse is not necessarily the diagnosis, but rather the act. Focusing on the act as the source of monstrosity is a potentially slippery slope. What counts as a monstrous act is not set in stone; monstrosity depends on the definer and the defined. If one act can be easily understood as horrible, tragic, and unspeakable, then many more acts can be described in much the same way. The risky mother identity is thus one that continues to constrain women's mothering practices, if only by the threat that any single act could become the next unacceptable behavior.

The issues of surveillance and monstrosity are precisely what undergird the disciplining of mothers who step outside (indeed, live outside) the boundaries of postfeminist motherhood; that is, women of color, single mothers, mothers on welfare, and so forth. That these two elements now also play fundamental roles in normalizing postpartum depression should give us pause. Consider, for example, the disciplining of women of color during the crack-baby crisis of the 1980s. According to Drew Humphries, media coverage of the use of crack by pregnant women inflamed a variety of stereotypes about "lower class sexuality and reproduction."[127] Black inner-city women were routinely depicted as feeling "indifferent to their suffering newborns."[128] Many states criminalized the use of drugs by pregnant women by using existing child endangerment laws, and poor black women were arrested and punished at a rate that was far higher than that of middle- and upper-class white women. Although states punished black mothers who used crack cocaine while pregnant, white women were routinely not punished for similar offenses such as using powder cocaine while pregnant. As this example illustrates, an act is never just an act; it always exists in a social context and is given meaning through larger discourses of (in this case) risky versus monstrous mothers, medical diagnoses, and the criminal justice system.

I have argued elsewhere that one of the problems of using wealthy white women to represent the face of postpartum disorders is that it gives white women access to the language of diagnosis and the promise of medical treatment for their behaviors while withholding these resources from women of color and women of lower socioeconomic status.[129] Discourses of surveillance and self-regulation that help normalize postpartum depression through the bodies and lives of elite white women condone their risky behavior (except for the final act of harming and/or killing their children), but this discourse leaves mothers who fall outside the risky mothering model open to closer scrutiny and discipline. In her analysis of several postpartum psychosis cases, Jane Huckerby recognizes this dual logic by describing how white mothers are often offered the label "mad," while mothers of color are labeled "bad." Such dual positioning of mothers preserves what Huckerby describes as the white, middle class "maternal myth" by focusing on white mothers' mental illnesses as individual biological problems that can be treated.[130] Where self-surveillance and surveillance by others is constructed as empowerment for white women, for "other" women, it is anything but empowering.

Critiquing the Institution of Motherhood:
The Experiences of Postpartum Fathers

The normalization of postpartum depression continues the process of ignoring the systemic sources of difficulties for new mothers. This point might seem counterintuitive, as the construction of postpartum depression as an acceptable medical phenomenon exists within a narrative of risky motherhood in which some of the problems of mothering are voiced quite frequently. However, the risky mother's voicing of her everyday problems—her anger when her children do not behave, her fear that she might hurt them, her desire to find some time for herself—rarely moves the discourse about postpartum depression (and motherhood broadly) past a focus on the individual woman. This focus on the individual is not quite the same thing as what feminist postpartum self-help advocates have attempted to draw attention to. As Taylor notes, women within feminist self-help organizations sought to bring to light the "heavy demands on modern mothers" and call attention to "the way that maternal self-sacrifice undermines women's identities and well-being."[131] Such groups then used feminism as a resource for "calling institutions to account for sustaining, reproducing, and legitimating the centrality of women's positions as mothers."[132] Feminist research on postpartum depression emphasizes the social context of mothering as one of the primary factors that causes distress during the postpartum period. Within the postfeminist narrative of risky motherhood, larger critiques of institutions and systems are difficult to find. As postfeminist subjects, risky mothers are silenced in their critique of the larger system, and the acceptance of a medicalized understanding of postpartum disorders is, in part, evidence of such a silence. Medical understandings of postpartum depression, after all, do not require a (re)consideration of the role of motherhood in U.S. society as a source of women's distress beyond a general understanding that motherhood requires women to make some adjustments to their new state.

What might finally bring sustained attention to the social context of mothering and perhaps to critiques of that social context is fatherhood. Fathers' roles as parents are changing in the United States. Although they are not as prevalent as blogs, memoirs, and fictional works about motherhood, works about modern fatherhood detailing the ups and downs of raising children are easy to find (see, for example, Michael Lewis's recent best seller *Home Game*). The attention to fatherhood has brought to light a finding that is not surprising: fathers get postpartum depression, too; estimates suggest that about one in ten new fathers experiences some form of depression. When fathers are the ones with postpartum depression, it becomes more difficult to craft an entirely biological explanation. This is not to say that biology disappears entirely. Dr. Richard Friedman notes that "like motherhood, fatherhood has its own biology, and it may actually change the brain."[133] He continues, "There is some evidence that testosterone levels tend to drop in men during their partner's pregnancy, perhaps to make expectant fathers less aggressive and more likely to bond with their newborns."[134] The irony cannot escape feminist readers: men are now victims of their hormones as well.

Despite the occasional foray into hormonal explanations, however, explanations that echo—word for word, topic for topic—the reasoning of feminist psychologists are more common. According to one psychologist, fathers "today are more involved in rearing children than ever, [but] they often lack the broad social networks enjoyed by mothers."[135] This psychologist points to one of the many issues that feminist psychologists have focused on for new mothers: the need for social support networks. Fathers echo the accounts of new mothers who point to substantial sleep disruption as a key factor in their postpartum distress. As reporter Liz Szabo writes, "Rahul Parikh says even his training as a pediatrician didn't adequately prepare him for those first few months of fatherhood. Unlike medical interns, who take turns working 24-hour shifts, parents never get a night off."[136] Parikh goes on to explain, "At home, when the baby screams, it's all on you."[137] Other accounts of fathers with postpartum depression point to identity changes and the loss of old identities. Joel Schwarzburg offers this explanation: "I love my son dearly, but when he was born—to my eyes, an oozy bundle of constant need—it felt as if I had traded in my own life in exchange. I expected parental pride to hit me like a recovered memory, but all I felt was loss. To his parent's eyes, the child never ages, so the loss felt like a permanent condition, eventually mutating into resentment."[138] Schwarzburg and Parikh's descriptions are uncannily similar to the words of women with postpartum depression. Armstrong titled one chapter of her book "Her Screamness Who Screams a Lot While Screaming"—a reference to her daughter's unending and very vocal demands.

Ultimately, public discourse about postpartum depression for fathers sees multiple factors at work; although hormones may play a role, so do many other social factors. Psychiatrist Irene Levine points to lack of sleep, added responsibilities, and economic stressors.[139] This focus on multiple factors has begun to affect the discourse about postpartum depression in women. According to the researcher heading one study of major postpartum depression in fathers, we should not be surprised that fathers also become depressed because they are subject to the same stressors as mothers: "feelings of stress and anxiety associated with fatigue, lack of sleep, changes in the marital relationship and concerns about finances and work."[140] More significantly, some discussions have begun to move the conversation about depression to structural issues. Rosemary Black reports that "researchers think the reason the United States has such a high risk for parental postpartum depression is because of such short parental leaves; a three-month maternity leave is standard here."[141] Psychologist Bruce Dolin's reflections on his own experiences also point to external, systemic factors: "I'm sure that if we hadn't been broke, and facing very short maternity leave for my wife (and virtually none for me), we might have all been calmer about dealing with a profound lack of sleep!"[142]

The idea that analysis of postpartum depression in men might prompt the kind of focus on social issues of parenting feminist activists desire is somewhat ironic. I should note, however, that it is not the only source of nonbiological (or at least multifactorial) explanations for the emotions and behaviors that are medically framed as postpartum depression. A growing movement of women and men who have adopted children also challenges the strict biomedical model. Laurie Tarkan describes the situation of one adoptive mother: "She felt overwhelmed by the round-the-clock demands of the baby. She experienced anxiousness, had bouts of weepiness and felt somewhat isolated and lost."[143] Adoptive mothers experience the same high expectations regarding mother-hood, but, as Tarkan notes, "cannot explain their symptoms by a drop in estro-gen levels."[144] However, as long as the cause of distress during the postpartum period continues to be framed as primarily medical, women—and perhaps now men—will seek solutions to the difficulties of parenting in the medical arena (including pharmaceutical drugs) instead of seeking larger systemic changes such as expanded maternity and paternity leave.

Chapter 4

The Postfeminist Concession

Young Women, Sex, and Paternalism

In the spring of 2007, headlines across the United States noted an emerging women's health controversy. A *New York Times* headline declared "Furor on Rush to Require Cervical Cancer Vaccine," and the *Dallas Morning News* offered this depiction of the issue: "Preventing Cancer or Promoting Sex?"[1] Most articles focused on the question at the heart of the controversy: Should the newly approved and heavily marketed "cervical cancer vaccine," Gardasil, be mandated for adolescent girls even though it also protects against human papillomavirus (HPV), a sexually transmitted disease? The state of Texas led the campaign for mandatory vaccination, under a direct executive order from Governor Rick Perry. His order required young girls to receive the new vaccine before entering the sixth grade and made Texas the first state to enact a mandate, but with the help of WIG (Women in Government, a group of women state legislators partially funded by Merck, Gardasil's creator), many states began the process of reviewing bills that would mandate the vaccine. Public health officials and some women's health advocates supported the mandate in Texas. They argued that a mandate was the best way to ensure equal access to the vaccine, a priority given the long-standing disparity in health issues related to cervical cancer (in the United States, both the incidence of cervical cancer and mortality rates are higher in nonwhite racial groups and women of lower socioeconomic status).[2] Monica Casper and Laura Carpenter explain the potential benefit of mandating the vaccine: "If vaccines are required for school-children and are included in government schedules, then third-party payers will be more likely to reimburse for vaccination, and public payers must ensure widespread coverage."[3]

The supporters of the Gardasil mandate met fierce and immediate opposition. By the time thirty-one state legislatures were considering mandating the vaccine in 2007, criticism had risen from groups across the political spectrum: "These strange bedfellows included Christian conservatives and their abstinence-only ilk, who have long argued that safe sex encourages profligate sex; a slew of Big Pharma critics, who see how Merck (which stands to make four billion dollars a year on the vaccine by most estimates) is angling to corner this huge new vaccine market; the growing antivaccine movement, which objects to all such school-entry requirements; the parental-rights folks with a libertarian strain, who bridle at any mandates regarding their children's health; and a smattering of women's health advocates, who worry that the pace of the vaccine's introduction is jeopardizing its ultimate success."[4] The outcry over state mandates of Gardasil led the Texas state legislature to reverse Governor Perry's executive order, and mandate legislation across the country was either withdrawn or failed in legislatures. As of summer 2010, only two legislatures had successfully enacted mandates (both with significant opt-out clauses): Washington, D.C., and Virginia.

In this chapter, I focus on one aspect of the controversy about mandating Gardasil: the sexuality of adolescent girls. This was certainly not the only aspect of the controversy, but it was a pivotal aspect in terms of the construction of identities for young women. At least three different groups offered depictions of HPV and cervical cancer during the controversy: the marketing campaign for Gardasil, the supporters of the mandate, and the opponents of the mandate. My analysis focuses on the interplay between the two spheres of public discourse in which these three voices existed—commercial discourse (the Gardasil marketing campaigns) and noncommercial discourse (news coverage and blogs that offered arguments for and against the mandate). I analyze three stages of the discourse: Gardasil's first marketing campaign, "One Less"; noncommercial constructions of the at-risk/risky young woman; and Gardasil's second campaign, "I Chose." I argue in my analysis that the risk of cervical cancer is superseded by the moral and physical risks of sex for a specific group of privileged young women. Through a confluence of postfeminist and paternalistic discourses, the *at-risk/risky young woman* is partially empowered in the medical sphere—when she is old enough, she can protect herself from the risk of cancer by choosing the vaccine—but she is disempowered in terms of her sexuality.

The emergence of paternalism as a factor in HPV/cervical cancer discourse can be related to several factors, including the age of the target audience for Gardasil. Although the vaccine was approved by the FDA in October 2006 for women ages nine to twenty-six, medical experts agree that it is most efficacious when given to women before they have been exposed to HPV. In pragmatic terms, this means that the vaccine is most effective before women have sexual experiences. Thus, Gardasil was originally marketed and the mandates were created with the lower half of the age spectrum as a target. In noncommercial discourse, these young women are typically identified as daughters who are in need of protection, not autonomous women who can mitigate risks through consumption of medical services or control over their sexuality. The interaction between the postfeminist and paternalist narratives points to postfeminism's easy alignment with traditional gender politics.

The Politics of Health Disparities and the Stigma of Sex

Globally, cervical cancer is the second most common cause of cancer-related death in women. Women in the global South ("resource-poor" areas such as Africa, Central America, and South America) constitute the majority of cases.[5] Using data from 2002, Eliav Barr and Heather Sings report that "cervical cancer has a disproportionate impact on women in developing countries[,] who account for about 85 percent of both yearly cases of cervical cancer (estimated at 493,000 cases worldwide) and the yearly deaths of cervical cancer (estimated at 273,500 cases worldwide)."[6] Women in the United States account for a small proportion of the global epidemic: in 2006 the United States had an estimated 9,710 cases of invasive cervical cancer and 3,710 deaths.[7] However, even in the United States, rates of incidence and mortality are related to race, ethnicity, and socioeconomic status.[8] According to Shobha Krishnan, Hispanic women have the highest incidence of cervical cancer. The incidence of the disease among African American women follows the rate among Hispanic women closely, but more African American women than Hispanic women die from the disease. Both Hispanic women and African American women have incidence rates substantially higher (more than 50 percent) than those of Caucasian women.[9]

These statistics point at least implicitly to the troubling status of cervical cancer as an example of global inequalities in access to health care that exist in part because only "a tiny proportion of the resources of our new biomedical era are directed to the major health problems of the majority of the world's population."[10] I include African American women, Hispanic women, and other groups of women of color in the United States as examples of global inequalities because, as Chandra Talpade Mohanty notes, they are part of an imagined community of "Third World women."[11] An important part of the history of cervical cancer is the history of exactly how cervical cancer became a problem for women in resource-poor settings but not for women in resource-high settings. In the 1960s, cytology screening, more commonly known as the Pap smear, became a routine part of women's health care in developed countries. Although not perfect (Pap smears are unable to detect all abnormalities), regular screening using the Pap smear led to a substantial drop in mortality from cervical cancer in developed countries.[12] However, cytology screening requires infrastructure (trained providers and technicians, adequate collection procedures, laboratories) that many developing countries do not have. From the beginning, cytology screening was a technology that only privileged women could access. Ultimately, the desire to develop an HPV vaccine was based in part on the "frustration that so many women in developing countries were dying from a preventable disease."[13] However, Carpenter and Casper remind us that before we unquestioningly embrace the potentially positive aspects of a HPV vaccine for women (in both developing and developed countries), the vaccine has been "introduced into a clinical, cultural, and geopolitical landscape profoundly shaped by modernist yet shifting notions of sex, gender, embodiment, contagion, health, progress and empire."[14] Such a complicated landscape suggests that the meaning of the vaccine (and indeed of cervical cancer) is contested terrain.

Two issues should give critical health scholars pause. The first is directly related to the vaccine's potential to reduce the disparities in the incidence of and mortality from cervical cancer among resource-poor and resource-high women. Carpenter and Casper explain: "'Postcolonial' practices of technology distribution and use for women's health may improve statistics—a goal of governmentality—but they may also replicate such misguided historical interventions as eugenic population-control programs or experimentation on poor women of color."[15] Cervical cancer prevention in developing countries is infused with problematic power dynamics; the World Health Organization offers different recommendations for cervical cancer screening based on a country's resources level (cytology screening for middle-income countries, visual cervical examination and acetic acid washing to detect lesions in lower-income countries, and HPV-DNA testing in countries with the requisite laboratory facilities). The ethics of the WHO's position—different screening policies for countries with different resource levels—is hotly debated.[16] Thus, women's access to medical care based on biomedical advances is shaped by where they live on the planet: "Women in resource-poor settings [are] defined differently from (and more pejoratively than) women in the global North."[17] Further, cervical cancer screening and prevention "activate cultural beliefs about gender and sexuality."[18] In Brazil, Pap smears have reinforced the belief that women's sexuality is dangerous and must be controlled, while in much of Africa and Asia, gynecological examinations are seen as a threat to women's sexual purity.[19] Although I have focused here on the global dimensions of postcolonial politics, many of the problems in terms of different expectations for and treatment of different groups of women are replicated at least partially in the United States.

The sexual politics surrounding cervical cancer generally and the HPV vaccine more recently constitute the second issue to which feminist scholars should be attuned. Even before the discovery of HPV in cervical cancer tissue in 1983, researchers had long suspected a link between cancer of the cervix and sexual activity. As early as the mid-nineteenth century, doctors were aware of the unique epidemiology of cervical cancer: women who had sex developed cervical cancer at far greater rates than women who remained celibate throughout their lives.[20] In a 1974 article, Valerie Beral suggested that it might be appropriate to understand cervical cancer itself as a sexually transmitted infection, noting that cancer of the cervix was "almost unknown in nuns" and that many factors that appeared to increase risk were related to sexual activity: marriage, broken marriage, multiple marriages, extramarital sexual activity, premarital sexual activity, early age of first marriage, early age of first intercourse, and multiple sexual partners of the woman and of the husband.[21] Without knowledge of HPV, practitioners developed a variety of other explanations for cervical cancer, placing the blame on smegma (which builds up under the foreskin of uncircumcised men who do not wash) in the 1950s and the herpes virus in the 1970s.[22]

The clear connection—made easily through epidemiological studies—between cervical cancer and sexual activity placed medical discussions of cervical cancer before the 1990s within larger cultural discussions of what was appropriate sexual behavior for women. In other words, unlike a cancer without a concrete connection between activity and risk (such as lymphoma), cervical cancer was from the beginning linked to lifestyle. And for women, a sexually active lifestyle, whether through marriage, multiple partners, or prostitution, is difficult discursive terrain. Underlying mid- to late twentieth-century medical discussions of cervical cancer were clear judgments about women's sexual activity and moral status. Virginia Braun and Nicola Gavey, who interviewed individuals who developed New Zealand's cervical cancer prevention policies, found that many informants reported negative perceptions of women with cervical cancer. One informant noted, for example, that it was common to hear statements indicating that "women who got cervical cancer were promiscuous. They were whores, sort of prostitutes."[23]

By the 1990s, the research on HPV and cervical cancer was making the connection between cervical cancer and women's sexual activity more concrete: "Cervical cancer was long considered to be just that, a cancer, and prevention and treatment proceeded accordingly. A major etiological shift occurred in the 1990s, and [cervical cancer] is now widely understood to be a sexually transmitted infection."[24] HPV is the most common sexually transmitted infection (STI) in the world (it is found throughout the human population), and it carries the stigma associated with sexually transmitted infections and diseases. Both men and women transmit and receive sexually transmitted infections, but women have long borne the brunt of the stigma associated with STIs. Adina Nack explains that STIs are often associated with a "blemish in character," and women are particularly vulnerable to the charge of promiscuity.[25] The stigma of STIs compounds the already restrictive and disciplining discourse about women's sexual behavior. Braun and Gavey explain: "STDs are employed to reinforce a dichotomy between sexually 'good' and sexually 'bad' women: The good girl is sexually responsible, has one (preferably spousal) sexual partner, and does not get STDs. The bad girl is sexually irresponsible, has many sexual partners, and gets STDs."[26]

Part of the gendered stigma of sexually transmitted infections could have been avoided or at least approached in a different manner if the two current HPV vaccines—Gardasil (approved by the FDA in October 2006) and Cervirax (approved in October 2009)—had received a gender-neutral approval from the FDA. Gardasil protects against four common types of HPV: types sixteen and eighteen, which are thought to cause about 75 percent of cervical cancer cases, and types six and eleven, which are connected to 90 percent of cases of genital warts.[27] Gardasil was approved by the FDA through a priority hearing that focused almost entirely on female bodies, although Merck had hoped from the beginning to secure approval for both girls and boys.[28] The director of the drug trials, Dr. Eliav Barr, made this clear in the hearing: "The ages we chose were those ages that would benefit most from administration of a prophylactic HPV vaccine, girls and boys age 9 to 15 and 16–26-year-old adolescent young women."[29] Although the vaccine can protect both men and women from specific strains of HPV, in the FDA trial it was understood as a preventative against cervical cancer, despite the goals of Merck and the researchers closely associated with the drug trials. This understanding of the vaccine is clearly at odds with Dr. Barr's description of the breadth of the vaccine's abilities: Gardasil "covers 70 of anal cancer, 70 percent of other HPV related cancers, 65 percent of pre-cancer transmission in men, 90 percent [of] genital warts, 90 percent [of] RRP [recurrent respiratory papillomatosis] lesions and transmission to women."[30]

The paradox that emerged from the FDA hearings—vaccinate women for a disease transmitted and received by both sexes—presented HPV as a women's health issue instead of a gender-neutral public health issue. By labeling HPV a women's health issue, the FDA's approval of Gardasil replicated the longstanding tradition of making women responsible for matters of sexual and reproductive importance.[31] Indeed, Gardasil entered the market as a gendered technology that was always already immersed in what Paula Treichler calls the "burdens of history" regarding women and sexually transmitted diseases.[32] This history in the United States includes the campaigns against venereal disease during the two world wars in which women were positioned as deceitful carriers and transmitters of disease who were poised to undermine U.S. war efforts by infecting young soldiers.[33] Merck's attempts to avoid the burdens of history regarding women and sexuality backfired, and the Gardasil girl of the "One Less" campaign was transformed into the sexually vulnerable young woman in noncommercial discourse.

Postfeminism and the Gardasil Girl

In late 2006, Merck launched the "One Less" marketing campaign for Gardasil. Most media commentators recognize the success of the "One Less" campaign in branding Gardasil. Merck and the "One Less" campaign also received numerous awards from the pharmaceutical industry.[34] *Pharmaceutical Executive* writer Beth Herskovits offered this glowing assessment: "By combining innovative science, strategic commercialization, and savvy disease education, Team Gardasil created a campaign that evoked Merck in its prime—and made strides toward stamping out cervical cancer."[35] Much of the power of the "One Less" campaign comes from the postfeminist narrative it spins about adolescent girls and their health. The FDA requires advertisements for pharmaceutical drugs to include specific content regarding safety and side effects, but advertisements also tell the public a story about the medication and those who take it.[36] The narrative of the postfeminist Gardasil girl in the "One Less" campaign of 2006 and 2007 offers a very specific meaning for the both the vaccine and those who use it: Gardasil is a vaccine that empowered, privileged adolescents choose to use to protect themselves against the risk of cervical cancer.[37]

The Privileged, Postracial Gardasil Girl

The narrative of the Gardasil girl in the "One Less" commercials is relatively straightforward. The commercials feature adolescent girls (sometimes with their mothers, but as often by themselves) engaging in a variety of everyday activities and declaring their desire to be "One Less" cervical cancer statistic. This is a narrative about maintaining health by recognizing risk (one commercial reminds us, "Each year in the United States thousands of women learn they have cervical cancer") and acting to prevent that risk.[38] Although at times the two primary advertisements I analyze are somber in tone, overall the narrative is cheerful; the adolescents who are declaring "I want to be one less" are moving toward a happy future free of cervical cancer.

At the center of the postfeminist narrative of the Gardasil girl is the Gardasil girl herself. This identity revolves around a key characteristic that unites what *Bitch* magazine describes as the "veritable rainbow" of youngsters that populate the commercial: postracial privilege.[39] Postracial discourse works in much the same way as postfeminist discourse; where postfeminist discourse presumes that women have reached full equality, postracial discourse presumes the disappearance of racism. Sumi Cho argues that under a postracialist ideology, "race does not matter, and should not be taken into account or even noticed."[40] Postracial discourses, including those that purport to be color blind or multicultural, draw our attention away from existing racism.[41] For the Gardasil girl, racial/ethnic backgrounds do not matter. The lived differences between racial/ethnic groups—specifically those differences related to disparities in health—are rendered largely invisible as the adolescents of the Gardasil commercials are all capable of making the decision to be "one less" cancer statistic.

The "One Less" commercials occasionally touch upon the cultural aspects of race/ethnicity. This engagement is most clear through the depiction of adolescents participating in a variety of activities. For example, one of the "One Less" commercials features nine adolescent women, three of whom are visually identifiable as African American. These three women are participating in activities that are "culturally appropriate"—playing basketball, dancing in a step troupe, and skipping rope in a game known commonly as double dutch. Lisa Traiger explains that step dancing is "part body percussion and party poetry slam" and notes that it "has been popular for decades on the African American fraternity and sorority circuit."[42] White adolescents in this commercial are skateboarding, playing soccer, sewing, and taking nature walks with their mothers. That so much time is spent depicting young women in different situations suggests that for the Gardasil girl, race/ethnicity matters to the extent that it sometimes influences what activities she chooses. This representation of cultural diversity supports a broader postracial message in the commercials in which race does not matter in terms of empowerment. Each Gardasil girl is positioned as having both an equal risk of cervical cancer and equal access to the vaccine. This message, of course, evades the different rates of cervical cancer among racial groups, an evasion that is supported by class privilege in the commercials. Put another way, class is a unifying factor in the Gardasil campaign's depiction of postracial womanhood.

The "One Less" campaign assumes that the postracial Gardasil girl will have easy access to the vaccine. This assumption is made clear both verbally and visually. A "One Less" commercial advises, "Ask your doctor about getting vaccinated with the only cervical cancer vaccine: Gardasil."[43] The African American adolescent appearing with her step troupe declares, "Gardasil does not prevent all types of cervical cancer so it is important to continue with routine cervical cancer screening."[44] Statements such as these are typical in direct-to-consumer advertisements that routinely urge the public to seek medical care, and the statements assume that medical care is readily available. In addition, the "One Less" commercials visually depict class privilege through the activities the Gardasil girls are participating in and the physical locations of the girls and their mothers. Many of the activities in the "One Less" commercials (including skateboarding, playing basketball, riding horses, drumming, playing soccer, driving in the country, going on nature walks, step dancing, sewing, painting, boxing, and playing double dutch) require money and middle-class status. The white adolescent who is skateboarding, for example, owns a skateboard and is skating in a skate park. The white mother/daughter pair depicted on a country drive are using a digital camera (they are taking photographs as they walk) and are driving a clean and modern four-door sedan. The horseback rider has access to a horse and riding equipment.

Some of these activities clearly signal middle-class status, but others—and I include playing double dutch in this category—are more ambiguous. The African American Registry, a nonprofit organization, describes double dutch as an activity "played by black children (mainly girls) in rural and urban areas in America."[45] It is associated in popular culture with urban America and with lower socioeconomic status. However, the Gardasil advertisements place the African American Gardasil girls playing double dutch in a middle-class context. Middle class is signified in this case by what it is not—bleak poverty or ostentatious wealth. The three adolescents playing double dutch are standing on a sidewalk in front of two row houses. The homes are similar in style and shape: both are painted gray, and both have porches and several front windows. One home has a staircase with white-painted wrought-iron railings. Between the two houses are manicured shrubs, and a potted plant sits on one porch. The sidewalk is broad and expansive. Standing out starkly against the light gray of the homes and the white of the sidewalk are three African American adolescents who are wearing black pants, green shirts, and white tennis shoes.

The visual message sent by the physical location of the adolescents is complex. The background for this activity aligns well with popular ideas of where the activity of double dutch might take place: the homes are not suburban ranch houses or "McMansions." The urban feel to the location, however, is combined with visual cues to middle-class status—the houses are well taken care of, the sidewalk is clean, the bushes are trimmed. These are homes, not merely houses, and they sit behind a sidewalk that is large enough to accommodate a double dutch game. The uniformly clothed adolescents are not playing in the street. Differences in geographical locations—urban, suburban, rural—do not, in these advertisements, represent differences in class status.

Empowering the Gardasil Girl

The privileged, postracial adolescents are empowered in a very specific and postfeminist way in the Gardasil girl narrative. Bree Kessler and Summer Wood of *Bitch* magazine describe the Gardasil girl as "savvy, self-aware, and rebellious," a girl who gives voice to a "feminist-lite rhetoric of consumer 'choice' as a form of empowerment for women"[46] As a *New York Times* writer explains, she is "the coolest girl in the room" and, for mothers, "our dream daughters . . . free but not reckless; strong but not angry."[47] These two reflections on the adolescents in the "One Less" campaign point to two specific iterations of empowerment: medical choice and agency, even as a daughter. The Gardasil girl's ability to choose to vaccinate and her role as an adolescent who is "free"—that is, one who has a certain degree of independence from her mother and other family members—are linked by an overarching theme of postfeminist girl power.

Both of the nationally aired commercials in the "One Less" campaign begin with a description of cervical cancer risk. The commercials report that cervical cancer develops from a common virus, HPV. Gardasil, they explain, protects against four types of HPV: "two types that cause 70 percent of cervical cancer, and two more types that cause other HPV diseases."[48] However, there is no acknowledgment of what other diseases might be attached to HPV. Further, there is no discussion of the details how the HPV virus operates, most pertinently how it is transmitted. Audiences are instead informed that the vaccine protects against the "human papillomavirus that may cause 70 percent of cervical cancer." This careful construction of HPV as a virus of unknown origin and the emphasis on cervical cancer sidestep discussions of sex. The Gardasil web site followed the emphasis on cervical cancer in 2006 and 2007, explaining that Gardasil was the only vaccine that could help guard against three health issues: cervical cancer, cervical abnormalities that can sometimes lead to cervical cancer, and genital warts.[49] Although the web site mentions genital warts, there is no discussion of HPV as a sexually transmitted disease on the first page, and genital warts is consistently listed as a secondary concern. Clicking on the "How is HPV transmitted" link brings up a page about sexual activity, but the term "sexually transmitted" is avoided.[50]

Because the risk adolescents face is defined specifically as cervical cancer and discussions of how HPV is transmitted are limited (in the commercials, not present at all), the only option given to the Gardasil girl for mitigating the risk is vaccination. The "One Less" commercials feature messages of empowerment that are typical in direct-to-consumer advertisements for pharmaceutical drugs: they declare "Ask your doctor about getting vaccinated with the only cervical cancer vaccine: Gardasil," and at the end of each commercial the words "GET VACCINATED" appear. The Gardasil girls are depicted as eagerly accepting and acting on this message. The adolescents playing double dutch incorporate the "One Less" slogan by chanting "O-N-E-L-E-S-S I want to be one less" as they skip rope. A young white woman literally labels herself "One Less" by stitching the words onto her hooded sweatshirt.[51] Consumption is a typical mode of empowerment for neoliberal subjects. However, something more than simple neoliberal empowerment through choice is happening as the adolescents take up the "One Less" motto. The middle-class activities the girls engage in play a role in crafting a girls' version of postfeminist empowerment that includes their choice to become vaccinated. In this way, the ads strongly imply, vaccination is just one more daily activity for these girls. But the subtext also conveys that vaccination is empowering in the same way that the activities they are doing are empowering. Although some of the adolescents are seen taking part in gender-typical activities (sewing, skipping rope), many of them are engaging in activities that have only recently become open to women: skateboarding, boxing, and playing soccer and basketball. Seen through the lens of girls playing sports formerly available to or culturally acceptable for men only, Gardasil is framed as an expression of the cultural phenomenon of girl power, which, as Marnina Gonick explains, configures adolescent girls in a particular way: they are "assertive, dynamic, and unbound from the constraints of passive femininity."[52] Although girl power has many roots and many iterations, its cooptation by the mass media, educational programs, and pop music has resulted in at least one consistent message: female achievement is based not in feminism but on female individualism.[53] For the Gardasil girls the choice to become vaccinated is an enactment of postfeminist girl power: a "gentle, non-political, and non-threatening" alternative to feminist empowerment.[54]

The Gardasil girl's ability to act on her own—as an assertive, autonomous, neoliberal subject—is emphasized in the advertisements even when her mother is present. In one "One Less" advertisement, only three of the nine adolescents who have speaking roles are linked with mothers. Thus, the majority of girls appear without their mothers. Furthermore, even those girls with their mothers are depicted as subjects with agency. In two of the three cases, the girls are engaged in activities (horseback riding and soccer) that reduce the mothers to spectators. In the third example, an adolescent and her mother are depicted on a nature walk. This is the only example in this advertisement of an adolescent and her mother in continuous contact with each other. The mothers' role in the "One Less" campaign is best characterized as a helpful spectator. All three mothers have speaking roles, and they are responsible for giving some of the clinical information about Gardasil, but the adolescents provide similar information. For example, the adolescent stitching "One Less" on her hooded sweatshirt informs the viewer that "Gardasil will not treat cervical cancer."[55] The adolescents are offered by far the most active role in the advertisements: they offer medical information, receive medical information, and (are expected to) act on that medical information. Although the mothers are occasionally present and convey some information, the adolescent girls are the ones directly depicted as wanting to be "One Less," and adolescent girls are clearly spoken to in the final acts of the commercials: the verbal message "With Gardasil, *you* could be one less" is followed by the order "Get Vaccinated."[56] The choice to become vaccinated rests with the Gardasil girl, although the mother's presence hints at the need for adult assistance to gain access to the vaccine.

Sex, Postracial Politics, and the Gardasil Girl Narrative

The choice of the privileged, postracial Gardasil girl to get vaccinated is aligned with a larger postfeminist girl-power discourse in which assertiveness and self-management is signaled through not only getting the vaccination but also their participation in an ever-expanding set of activities and their independence from their mothers. The narrative in the ad campaign defuses at least two potential stumbling blocks in terms of marketing the vaccine. First, and most importantly, constructing the risk of HPV as a risk of cancer not only places Gardasil in larger positive discourses about preventing cancer but also enables Merck to negotiate the very tricky ground of selling a vaccine for a sexually transmitted disease to young women and their parents (most often their mothers) by avoiding discussions of sex for the most part. Cultural understandings of youth and sexuality in the United States focus on the idea of sexual innocence. In practical terms, this is often combined with a "conviction that youth are highly suggestible, easily 'infected' by all manner of potentially undesirable behaviors."[57] Many politicians, parents, and policymakers who attempt to "curb young people's activities by controlling access to sexual information in mass media and schools" subscribe to the theory that young people are "sexually innocent but easily suggestible."[58] Assumptions about youth and sexuality inform many attempts to prevent youth from any access to information about sex. The construction of cervical cancer as the primary risk women face in terms of HPV infection attempts to avoid the problem of sex by displacing it with a concern for cancer, a universally feared disease.

Not surprisingly, Merck's attempt to avoid linking their vaccine to sex does not prevent discussions of sex and young women's sexuality in noncommercial public discourse. Part of this failure is based on the different exigencies politicians and Merck face. A second reason is related to the issue that because of its explicit use of the virus's name—human papilloma virus, HPV—in its advertisements, Merck is unable to completely avoid the specter of sex. Merck never seeks to "un-name" the virus that causes cervical cancer. In its earliest marketing campaign, "Tell Someone" (which aired before Gardasil was approved by the FDA), Merck identifies the virus as HPV. The "Tell Someone" campaign was aimed at helping women make the connection between HPV and cervical cancer, a connection that was mostly unknown to the public.[59] In the campaign's advertisements, no mention is made of Gardasil, but women (including mothers with their daughters) are depicted as expressing surprise at the prevalence of HPV: "I was stunned at how many people have HPV. I was stunned. Millions? That's insane."[60] Various women then face the camera directly to instruct audiences to "tell someone" of the viral connection to cancer. Again, because it makes no mention of methods of transmission (the virus is simply framed as common), Merck attempts to avoid discussions of sex and sexuality. However, the success of this evasion depends on the audience's lack of information about the HPV virus. This ignorance worked in Merck's favor in its desire to avoid discussions of sex. In a national study of focus groups published in 2007, Allison Friedman and Hilda Shepeard confirm the low level of knowledge about HPV. For example, focus group participants identified genital warts as a sexually transmitted infection but rarely mentioned HPV.[61] Women were slightly more likely to have heard about HPV (from friends, gynecologists, and magazines), but out of the 314 people in the focus groups, only 3 knew of the connection between HPV and cervical cancer.[62] The lack of knowledge about HPV suggests that much of Merck's audience may very well not have been aware of HPV's status as a sexually transmitted infection. Thus, at least initially, Merck's "Tell Someone" public awareness campaign and the later "One Less" campaign were at least partially successful in presenting the vaccine as unrelated to sex and the stigma of STIs.

Second, the careful construction of privileged, postracial adolescents in the Gardasil girl narrative flattens the complex social context of cervical cancer and cervical cancer screening. Most pertinently, in the advertisements the adolescents featured are at universal risk of cervical cancer and have a universal ability to manage that risk. Critics of the "One Less" campaign have pointed to Merck's failure to address disparities in the health status of racial groups in its public messages. Sheila Rothman and David Rothman decry the lack of focus on populations at higher risk, including "populations in geographic areas with excess cervical cancer mortality, including African Americans in the South, Latinos along the Texas-Mexico border, and whites in Appalachia."[63] Merck's "One Less" campaign is, in their critique, not "risk-sensitive" and thus not necessarily targeted toward the populations that might benefit most from the vaccine.[64] My concern with Merck's construction of the Gardasil girl is related to the critique Rothman and Rothman offer: the deliberate use of adolescents from numerous racial/ethnic backgrounds offers the overly simple message that all adolescent girls are equally at risk of cervical cancer and that all adolescents should choose (and have the same ability to choose) to be vaccinated. Jessica Polzer and S. Knabe offer a similar critique in the Canadian context, arguing that Merck's advertisements "blur the line between public health education and the marketing of pharmaceutical products," focus on women's individual responsibility (and ability) to choose the vaccine, and obscure the "social conditions and determinants associated with higher rates of mortality from cervical cancer among marginalized women."[65] Unfortunately, the universalization of both the risk of and the responsibility for avoidance of cervical cancer is replicated (in a slightly different form) in noncommercial public discourse about cervical cancer.

Paternalism and the At-Risk/Risky Young Woman

By the time Governor Rick Perry released his executive order mandating the HPV vaccine for all girls entering the sixth grade in Texas, Gardasil's "One Less" campaign was a significant player in the construction of public understandings of the vaccine, HPV, cervical cancer, and women facing the risk of cervical cancer. News reports frequently turned to the "One Less" slogan to discuss cervical cancer, and the term "Gardasil girl" began to be used to describe young women who had received the vaccine. One approach to analyzing the relationship between Merck's advertisements and noncommercial public discourse is to understand Merck as an agenda setter. Broadly speaking, agenda setting refers to the "ability of a media organization or institution to determine the important issues for debate or consideration."[66] I am using the term to suggest that the advertisements for Gardasil attempted to set the terms for public noncommercial discussions about the vaccine. The agenda in this case was crafted through the Gardasil girl narrative and in response to a variety of problematic contextual factors, including the stigma of STIs. In my analysis of news coverage of the mandate controversy from 2006 to 2009, I argue that the public continued to work within at least part of this frame—the bodies and lives of privileged adolescents.[67] However, the "One Less" campaign was not successful in diverting attention away from sex.

Merck's ability to avoid sex is directly linked to their position as marketers of a specific pharmaceutical drug. Political figures—like the individuals who supported mandate legislation—had to discuss HPV's categorization as an STI as part of the mandate campaigns, in part because the mandates needed to include information about why the vaccine was appropriate for girls of a certain age. The mandate controversy that developed in the winter and spring of 2007 inevitably turned to discussions of sex because of the pragmatic constraints politicians face. Merck's choice to effectively cede discussions of sex to noncommercial actors relinquished the company's ability to shape the discussion of sex that did occur. In the rest of this chapter, I look at how sex, sexual activity, and sexuality in relation to HPV and cervical cancer was framed in the mandate controversy. I argue that in noncommercial discourse, discussions of HPV, cervical cancer, and sex developed through a paternalist narrative of protection that articulates a new identity for adolescents and young adult women: the at-risk/risky young woman. I develop this argument by analyzing the emergence of paternalism as a guiding frame in noncommercial discourse. The paternalist ideology of protection transforms the privileged, postracial Gardasil girl into a young woman facing the risks associated with sex.

Paternalism and Noncommercial Public Discourse

Paternalism has long played a role in discussions of women's health. Advocates in the women's health movement fought paternalist practices that deprived women of agency and autonomy in the medical arena. Kathy Davis offers this definition of paternalism: "[The] concept of power which combines the element of benevolence with the elements dominance and subordination. . . . it entails, by definition, limiting the freedom of another person by means of well-meant regulations. In this way, benevolent intentions are combined with relations of power. . . . Paternalism—again, by definition—implies a relationship of asymmetry. The original model for a paternalistic relationship is that of a parent and child."[68] Gender paternalism (based in a male-female hierarchy) replicates the parent-child dynamic by turning women "into children who need guidance."[69] Reva B. Siegel emphasizes that gender paternalism is often used to deprive women of legal agency, "rationalizing gender hierarchy in the discourse of protection."[70] The emergence of paternalism in discussions of HPV, cervical cancer, and sex can be linked to two trends in noncommercial public discourse that focus on privileged youth: limiting the discussion of health disparities to certain contexts and emphasizing the health and safety of "our daughters."

The focus on privileged adolescents in the "One Less" campaign carried over into noncommercial discourse, with one exception: actors in noncommercial discourse recognized that there was a potential disparity regarding access to the vaccine. Discussions about the broader disparities in the incidence of cervical cancer and mortality rates from that disease appear only rarely, and the strongest statements about health disparities occur in terms of the cost of the vaccine: $360 for the three-shot regimen.[71] Texas governor Rick Perry's executive order mandating the vaccine took the issue of cost into account, and the order included a mandate that the vaccine be made immediately available to low-income Texans through the Texas Vaccines for Children and Medicaid programs.[72] Concerns about price also appeared in national news coverage as justification for the mandate. The *New York Times* ended an editorial in support of the mandate with this statement: "A mandate would force the health system to get cracking. And it is the best way to ensure that all children get the vaccine, not just those who are aware of it and can afford it."[73] However, very few articles tackled the complexity of health disparities beyond the issue of access to the vaccine. In the United States, cervical cancer morbidity and mortality rates are stratified by race and ethnicity and socioeconomic status for many reasons, including but not limited to differences in access to health insurance, differences in knowledge about and attitudes toward cervical cancer and sexually transmitted infections, and the systems of inequality (including those of race, class and gender) that shape the "ideological, political, and economic domains of society in institutional structures and in individual lives."[74] Ultimately, in public discourse health disparities are reduced to a discussion of whether or not a population has access to the vaccine, and even that discussion occurs in limited and infrequent contexts. The issue of access became the final justification for a mandate after a long series of arguments about the vaccine.

The reduction of the many health disparity issues involved with the Gardasil vaccine to one of access is part of the larger trend of focusing on postracial, privileged adolescents like the girls that were featured in the Merck campaign rather than on the complexity of the lived context of those with cervical cancer and all of the inequalities that context evokes.[75] Consistent calls in noncommercial discourse to "protect our daughters" are part of this trend. The term "our daughters" signifies a very raced and classed notion of womanhood. When used in public discourse, phrases such as "our daughters" and "our sons" often call forth the values of white, middle- and upper-class, heterosexual culture.[76] Arguments about the appropriateness for the vaccine for "our daughters" (and endless variations, including "our preteen girls" and "our teenage daughters") emerged almost immediately after the FDA approved Gardasil, but they gained strength after the Texas mandate passed, from groups that opposed and groups that supported the mandate. Suzanne M. Horn from The Woodlands (a wealthy Houston suburb) ended her letter to the editor of the *Houston Chronicle* with a plea to "support this vaccination. It can save our daughters' lives."[77] James Nelson of Austin made the following statement in the *Austin-American Statesman*: "I am outraged at the audacity of Perry to issue an executive decree to require our preteen girls to submit to inoculation with Merck's new scare drug."[78] In an article titled "Protecting Our Daughters," Penna Dexter suggested that "perhaps a sense of 'self worth' will protect our daughters from getting involved in the sexual behaviors that will only harm them."[79]

Although no extensive work was done in public discourse to specifically define "our daughters," that phrase and its various iterations work to centralize the privileged daughters who follow the values of white, middle-class America, whether they are white or not. In news coverage about the mandate, class was the defining difference between "our daughters" and other girls, replicating the importance of class in the construction of the postracial, privileged Gardasil girl. Consider, for example, a discussion about other daughters from the *Dallas Morning News*: "When you strip away all the huffy rhetoric about 'parental rights,' we're looking at a law that would have benefited the daughters of the least responsible parents. It would have addressed those girls from overburdened or dysfunctional households, the ones least able or likely to take voluntary extra measures to safeguard their children's health."[80] "Those girls," as the reporter refers to the underprivileged young women who need assistance to access to the vaccine, were not positioned in this article as "our daughters" or "our girls."

However, the privileged adolescents that were the focus of concern in mainstream discourse were positioned in a very different way than the Gardasil girl of the "One Less" campaign. Understood as "our daughters," the adolescents at the heart of the debate about the HPV vaccine mandate are not figures with agency; they are part of a larger family unit, whether that family unit is a nuclear family or the larger family of the state. Further, as daughters, the adolescents in noncommercial discourse take on a familial role that positions them at the bottom of the gender hierarchy. The paternalist urge to protect based on women's position in the nuclear and/or state family is clear, for example, in coverage of Rick Perry's executive order. In a speech given after the mandate was overturned by the state congress, Perry positioned himself as working for the protection of "our young women." His central motive, he said, "has been and always will be about protecting women's health."[81] As a protector, he believes in the benefit of mandating the vaccine because "even when young people are cautious . . . they could still become a victim of HPV."[82] The emergence of paternalism as a key frame in noncommercial discourse was thus tied to a specific construction of the adolescent girl and of women more broadly. She is "our daughter," an implicitly privileged figure who is constructed through a raced and classed discourse of traditional womanhood.

From the Gardasil Girl to the Young Woman

When paternalism rather than postfeminism is the lens through which adolescent girls and women are understood in noncommercial discourse, a distinctly different narrative develops. In the "One Less" campaign, the Gardasil girl is depicted as an autonomous subject, an individual who incorporates getting a vaccine against cancer into her many daily activities. Her choice to get the vaccine is easy to make, as she is assumed to have access to medical care and the financial resources to pay for the vaccine. As a mechanism of empowerment, receiving the

vaccination—like boxing, drumming, or playing basketball—solidifies her position as a consuming, postfeminist subject. The paternalist narrative that I explore
in this section and the next constructs a new subject position for adolescents:
the young woman. In this narrative, the young woman is positioned as vulnerable to a series of risks, but the primary risk is the risk of sex. Mitigating this risk
is the responsibility of her parents, not the young woman herself, although the
young woman continues to be held responsible for acts of sex, including rape
and incest. In this section, I analyze the young woman's relationship to her family, a key relationship given the paternalist frame of the narrative.

At the heart of the young woman identity are traditional gender expectations that reflect the young woman's status as a privileged, postracial figure. His-
torian Phyllis Marynick Palmer's discussion of "cult of true womanhood"—an
understanding of womanhood that developed in the nineteenth century for
white middle- and upper-class women—is useful here. She explicitly points to
how race and class often play a role in understandings of good and bad womanhood: "The symbolic division created in the nineteenth century was between
the 'good' women, who were pure, clean, sexually repressed, and physically
fragile, and the 'bad' women, who were dirty, licentious, physically strong,
and knowledgeable about the evil done in the world. Good women were wives,
mothers, spinsters—women dependent on men and sexually un-challenging.
Bad women were whores, laborers, single mothers—women who earned their
own bread and were politically and socially powerless. The dual symbolism of
good/bad was usually connected with race and class, but it could be used to
chastise any woman moving out of her assigned place."[83] The postracial class
privilege of the adolescent figure constructed in cervical cancer discourse eases
the process through which she moves from the empowered Gardasil girl to
the protected young woman. By using the specific term "young woman" as a
label for this new identity, I emphasize two dimensions of the larger paternalist
narrative: the young woman's current role as a daughter and her future roles
as wife and mother. The young woman is positioned as a good woman; she
is a "pure, clean, sexually repressed" woman whose future holds the roles of
wife and mother. She is also expected to participate in what Adrienne Rich
describes as compulsory heterosexuality: a political institution that disempow-
ers women by creating the assumption that women are innately sexually oriented toward men, thereby ensuring men the right to physical, economic, and
emotional access to women.[84]

From Empowerment to Protection: The Role of Mothers

Before a young woman becomes a wife and mother, she is first a daughter and thus a member of the family who is in need of protection. Unlike the mothers of the Gardasil advertisement, mothers in noncommercial discourse play an important role in protecting and making decisions for their daughters. Mothers were introduced in news coverage as individuals who have special insight into the vaccination controversy. The *Austin American-Statesmen* ended an article covering arguments against the mandate with this statement: "Marcela Contreras of South Austin, who has a 23-year-old daughter, said that if her daughter were younger, she would talk to her about not having sex before allowing her to get the vaccine."[85] Contreras's credibility comes directly from her position as a mother, and this credibility is used even when women have other sources of authority. Jane Nelson, a Texas state senator, is introduced this way: "state Sen. Jane Nelson, R-Lewisville, a critic of Perry's mandate and the mother of four daughters."[86] Mothers were highly visible in public discourse during this period: they were interviewed, quoted, and brought in as experts in discussions of whether or not to vaccinate their daughters.

Mothers in noncommercial discourse were only occasionally joined by fathers, who were given credibility specifically because of their position as parents. That mothers were more visible in this discourse than fathers may have been because the health issue affected women, but no matter which parent was speaking, the message from adults was the same: daughters need to be protected. One mother, a gynecologist living in Austin, explained her reason for giving the vaccine to her twelve- and fourteen-year-old daughters: "There are about a million things that my kids can do, a million mistakes they can make, that will mess up their lives, and I was able to take one away."[87] This mother's justification for giving her daughter the vaccine is the same as that of those who wish to avoid the vaccine: protection. However, unlike this mother, many parents (both those in support of the vaccine and those wary of the vaccine) focused on protecting their daughters not from cancer but from sex. Ultimately, both stances pivot on the understanding of the young woman as someone who is unable to make smart decisions and in need of guidance from others. In an editorial that supported a mandate for the HPV vaccine Alberta Phillips pointed to the paternalist undertones of the debate, "Social conservatives are fighting mad over Perry's order, which they assert promotes sexual promiscuity among teenagers and usurps parents in making decisions about their daughters."[88] Phillips, like the mother I discussed above, points to parents' belief in their right to make decisions for their daughters as one of the key factors in both resistance to and support for a vaccine mandate. As daughters, young women—unlike the Gardasil girls of the "One Less" campaign—have little autonomy in this coverage because they are seen to be in need of the protection and decision-making skills of the adults around them.

From Empowerment to Protection: The Future Roles of Young Women

The voices of concerned mothers in the noncommercial discourse serve another purpose. They are the future of young women: former daughters who are now mothers. Discussions about protecting young women's fertility were often used as a jumping point in noncommercial discourse to either support or work against the Gardasil mandate. Silvia Ford's story is an exemplar of this type of news coverage: "Silvia Ford, a 35-year-old stay-at-home mother from Maryland, learned in November 2004, just three months after bearing her second child, that she had cervical cancer. Surgeons removed her uterus, for which she has no regrets. 'I wanted to be around to take care of the two children I've already got.'"[89] Ford plays a dual role in this coverage. She is both a mother and a cervical cancer survivor, and she gives voice to one of the dangers cervical cancer poses: it takes mothers away from their children. As important, however, is what she says next: "This vaccine should not lead to an argument about when girls have sex. It's about saving the lives of women in their child-bearing years, letting them have children or take care of the children they already have."[90] Ford's argument gets to the heart of the matter: HPV can negatively affect not only a mother's ability to care for her children but also a potential mother's capacity to have children.

Anecdotes such as Ms. Ford's personalized the message about fertility and future motherhood, and they were used prolifically by Rick Perry in his mandate campaign. In his interviews and speeches in support of his executive order, Governor Perry offered several examples of women who were battling HPV. Two of his most striking examples returned the mandate fight to the setting of reproduction and domesticity. Perry explained why the HPV vaccine mandate was important: "And this is not some arcane policy debate. We're talking about real lives. Lives like Barbara Garcia, whose battle with cervical cancer now confines her to a wheelchair. She won't live to see her 9 year old son one day graduate from high school . . . or ask his sweetheart to marry him."[91] The lesson of Garcia's experience is similar to that of Ford: cervical cancer threatens motherhood. Perry also enlisted the story of Heather Burcham, a young woman who after five years of misdiagnosis found out that she had invasive cervical cancer. Perry concluded his final speech about his executive order by announcing that

Heather would have the last word, as "she has something to say, and I think it's infinitely more important than anything written in this bill."[92] In her video statement, Burcham was sitting in a bed wearing a white shirt with a vase of fresh pink tulips behind her. The thin, dark-haired Burcham explained how cancer had changed her life: "This cancer has taken from me the fact that one day I wanted to get married and I wanted Craig Wilson [a good friend and caretaker] to walk me down the aisle. I wanted to find my soul mate. And I wanted to have children. And because of this cancer that has been taken away from me and I can no longer have children which I wanted so badly."[93] Burcham died in 2007 at the age of thirty-one. Her narrative included descriptions of the pain she suffered on a daily basis and her desire to help others avoid cancer. Being heartbroken because of the realization that "getting married, having children, it was over" did not stop Burcham from attempting to spread the word about HPV. Burcham is the perfect depiction of a regretful young woman—the result of the transformation of the privileged, postfeminist Gardasil girl through paternalist discourses of protection and patriarchal expectations about womanhood. She would never have the chance to have children, and Burcham publicly mourned her lost future as wife and mother.

The Young Woman and Risk

The young woman of noncommercial discourse is an identity that resurrects key aspects of the discourse of true womanhood, including a focus on women's reproductive capacities and their roles as daughters and future mothers. Unlike the empowered Gardasil girl of the advertisements, the young woman is represented as vulnerable and in need of protection. The construction of the risk this young woman faces is directly linked to her identity as a (future) woman. Noncommercial discourse disrupts the postfeminist narrative about cervical cancer offered in the Gardasil commercials and replaces it with a narrative about young girls, sex, and morality. Because the young woman is constructed through a paternalistic lens discussions of sexuality begin with the premise that young women are in danger and need to be protected from sex. More specifically, young women need to be protected from heterosexual sex; sexuality outside of the heterosexual matrix is not included in the conversation that constructs the identity of the young woman. Sex is not just any risk; it is the most salient risk in noncommercial public discourse. This risk was constructed through two maneuvers in noncommercial discourse. First, both supporters and opponents of the mandate used a linear logic to describe the risk to young women that positioned sex as the first risk they encounter. Second, noncommercial discourse bifurcated the identity of the young woman into two dimensions of the good, sexually pure woman, the at-risk young woman and the risky young woman.

This linear logic is clear in the heated discussions about the actions young women engage in that lead to HPV. Rick Perry explains the necessity of vaccinating young women early: "Requiring young girls to get vaccinated before they come into contact with HPV is responsible health and fiscal policy that has the potential to significantly reduce cases of cervical cancer and future medical costs."[94] Perry and his supporters explained that young women come into contact with HPV through "sexual activity," but the fact that an activity (any activity) is the cause of the HPV transmission became a sticking point for many of those who opposed the mandate.[95] As Alan Katz wrote in a letter to the *New York Times*, "As desirable a thing as it may be to protect people from cervical cancer, a noncommunicable disease, it is a usurpation of government authority to dictate medical decisions that only individuals may make. Schools may rightfully require that children undergo immunizations that protect schoolwide populations from acquiring communicable diseases, but cervical cancer does not fall into this category."[96] Compared to other diseases for which vaccines exist (for example, the flu) that can be transmitted through the air, HPV and cervical cancer are positioned as transmissible through engagement in a specific set of activities. The linearity of the logic in some noncommercial public discourse about HPV and cervical cancer is present even without consideration of the sexual nature of the activity. According to this logic, a young woman must first act, and through her action, she increases the likelihood of contracting the virus. The virus can then lead to cancer. In this formulation of action that leads to virus that leads to cancer, it is the act itself that becomes the risk women face.

Theorists Barbara Adam and Joost van Loon argue that in the politics of risk, the definition of risk is always highly contested in terms of who is defining risk and how.[97] These contestations point to the very situated nature of knowledge about risk and suggest that knowledge of risk, which is created by pharmaceutical companies, politicians, parents, or even organizations such as Focus on the Family, privileges certain points of view. In noncommercial public discourse about HPV and cervical cancer, the fact that the act in question is sex (or any sexual activity that involves skin-to-skin genital contact) gives additional power to the linear logic, as sex is already understood—especially for young women who are not yet married—as a potentially dangerous act. The writer of one *New York Times* letter to the editor expanded the dangers of sexual activity for women beyond contracting HPV and getting cervical cancer to include "unplanned pregnancy, other sexually transmitted diseases, sexual assault, drug abuse, low self-esteem, boredom and depression."[98] Indeed, sex education programs to protect innocent youth from sex constitute a multimillion-dollar business. In abstinence programs, even "abstinence-plus" programs that offer some information on safe sex, "the privileging of abstinence over safer sex suggests that it is still unacceptable for educators to refrain from judging teens who choose to engage in risky sexual behavior, and tacitly concedes that abstinence is always a more legitimate and appropriate goal than safer sex."[99] In this cultural context, for "innocent youth" (a description that, as Jessica Fields notes, is never race or class neutral) sex is always dangerous, and the dangers range from physical to psychological.[100] In her comments about the Gardasil vaccine, Linda Klepacki of Focus on the Family, a conservative Christian group based in Colorado Springs, invokes the linear logic that places sex as the primary risk: "You can't catch the virus, you have to go out and get it with sexual behavior." She continues, "We can prevent it by having the best public health method, and that's not having sex before marriage."[101] Having sex means taking a risk, and in the linear logic both supporters and opponents of the mandate use, HPV and cervical cancer are only two in a long list of consequences for engaging in sex.

Within the linear logic of act-virus-cancer, sex becomes the beginning point of many of the discussions about preventing HPV/cervical cancer. However, within these discussions, it is the young women who are positioned as future wives and mothers who face the risks associated with sex. In noncommercial discourse, the young woman's relationship to sex works not only to disempower her in relation to her own sexual experiences, but also to reify her position as an essentially white—read postracial, privileged—subject. I do not mean that she is always Caucasian but rather that she conforms to hegemonic notions of proper sexual behavior and morality that are raced as white. The concern expressed about young women's sexuality emerges out of a concern for protecting the bodies and lives of pure women, of good women, and these women are always already configured as white. The construction of the young woman in relation to sex replicates the discussions of the sexual innocence of youth that occur in contemporary public discourse about abstinence-only sex education. As Jessica Fields notes, "Though notions of youthful sexual innocence and irredeemable sexual corruption may seem generic, they have a long-racialized history in the United States. Purity, sexual and otherwise, is routinely linked to whiteness, and, like low-income people, African Americans 'are generally excluded . . . from the privileging and protective invocation of innocence.'"[102] In the construction of the young woman, the focus on a postracial class privilege has made the "hypersexual bad girl"—a lower-class woman or a woman of color—invisible.[103] This is true in both noncommercial discourse and (implicitly) in the postfeminist Gardasil girl narrative of the "One Less" campaign. As an always already sexually pure character, the young woman faces the risk of sex from two positions: she is depicted as either at risk (a pure, good woman) or risky (a good woman on the verge of turning bad).

The at-risk young woman, the sexually pure and innocent adolescent, plays an important role in arguments for and against the mandate. For opponents of the mandate, the at-risk young woman is in moral danger because they believe that getting the vaccine may encourage young women to have sex. In fact, in early conversations, the HPV vaccine was dubbed the "promiscuity vaccine." In an article in the *Austin American-Statesman*, a person identified only as Adams, a representative of "conservative groups" protesting the mandate, noted: "Would they be more promiscuous? Chances are very good that they would be."[104] An Austin mother went so far as to suggest that just talking about the vaccine might encourage sexual activity: "There's always that feeling in the back of your mind any time you tell children about sex, or anything, that they're going to think that you're condoning it."[105] Leslee Unruh, president of the Abstinence Clearinghouse, offered a similar point of view: "Premarital sex is dangerous, even deadly. Let's not encourage it by vaccinating 10-year-olds so they think they're safe."[106] For opponents of the vaccine, sex is already configured as dangerous, and for young women it is morally dangerous. In their ideology, getting vaccinated actually heightens the risks the at-risk young woman faces instead of diminishing them. For this group, the concern about promiscuity takes precedence over concerns about HPV and cervical cancer. The specter of the morally compromised young woman, a woman whose reputation and standing in her community is questionable, looms as large as the threat of cervical cancer. The concern about promiscuity, of course, reflects the paradox of young women's sexuality: they are seen as pure and sexually innocent, but even good young women (with the slightest provocation) can become sexually dangerous and uncontrollable.[107]

Supporters of the mandate attempted to move the discussion away from issues of promiscuity, but the at-risk young woman was a central figure in their arguments too. One *New York Times* reporter asked, "Why would this vaccine give girls license to be sexually indulgent? It protects against only one sexually transmitted problem, and there are so many others, including Chlamydia, trichomoniasis, H.I.V. and, of course, unwanted pregnancy."[108] Pushing the promiscuity problem aside, supporters of the mandate focused on another issue: How does one justify a mandate for a vaccine that prevents a sexually transmitted disease when that mandate purports to target sexually innocent young women? The answer was found quickly and voiced by Perry and medical experts: young women cannot control their future husband's sexual activity and they certainly cannot hope to control the sexual behaviors of sexual predators. Perry embodied the problem in the story of a young woman, Amanda Vail, who was raped. Vail testified at the hearings about Gardasil in the Texas legislature after Perry's executive order. Explaining that her doctors had told her that she had a strain of HPV that could cause cervical cancer, she declared that she felt that she was injured anew by her attacker each time she had a Pap smear: "I would not have to be repeatedly violated had I been vaccinated."[109] Thus, as Perry explains, while society can "encourage young people to engage in monogamous behavior," they can still become victims of this "insidious virus" through rape.[110] Medical experts agreed with Perry's assessment. In the *New York Times*, journalist Denise Grady wrote, "Abstinence until marriage can prevent HPV infection, but is sure to work only if both spouses are virgins and remain monogamous forever." Grady quoted Laura Koutsky, a professor of epidemiology at the University of Washington in Seattle: "'You'd also have to guarantee—I hate to say it—that you're not going to be raped,' Dr. Koutsky said. 'If you're convinced that you can guarantee for your daughter that all those activities will or will not happen, then chances are good there will not be HPV transmission.'"[111]

The at-risk young woman is a highly vulnerable identity; she is vulnerable to the act of sex on many different levels. With the vaccine she will be protected from "external vulnerabilities"—the sexual actions of others. If she is raped, the vaccine will protect her from her assailant. But opponents of the mandate position the vaccine itself as increasing young women's vulnerability to moral disintegration. If offered the vaccine, the good young woman at the heart of the at-risk identity may be tempted to engage in promiscuous sexual behavior. Haunting this discussion of the good at-risk young woman is the figure of the risky young woman, the young woman who is already engaging (or could be engaging in the future) in risky behaviors (in this case, sex). The risky young woman is described from two vantage points. First, as I have suggested above, there is the potential that good at-risk young women will begin engaging in risky sexual behavior.

Second, the risky young woman emerges when advocates for the vaccine attempt to refute the concern about promiscuity by suggesting that just because a young woman is sexually active does not mean that she does not deserve the chance to be vaccinated and protected. From a feminist perspective, this line of argument has the potential to disrupt the good girl/bad girl dichotomy if there is also a recognition that sex for the young woman is in itself not morally wrong. However, this is not the path that noncommercial public discourse takes. Rick Perry offers the clearest version of the position of the risky young woman in public discourse:

> I therefore wholeheartedly reject the argument that this order encourages promiscuity, and even if I thought the argument had weight, I believe the greater imperative is to protect life. People do make wrong choices. But if we had a vaccine for lung cancer, would we discourage its availability because smoking is an inherently unhealthy activity? Where is our compassion for the health and well-being of our young women if we do not do all we can to protect each other from tremendous pain and suffering in the future? For all people of faith who, like me, are grateful for God's grace and forgiveness, how can we not respond with anything but compassion, grace, and forgiveness for those who may have fallen off the path of virtue at one point in their life?[112]

Sex is positioned in this example as something, like smoking, that is inherently unhealthy. Despite Perry's talk about compassion and forgiveness, risky young women are judged in this discourse. Peterson and Lupton point to one of the problems of focusing on lifestyle factors in public health discussions: "In the event that one is unable to regulate one's own lifestyle and modify one's risky behaviour, then this is, at least in part, 'a failure of the self to take care of itself.'"[113] In public discourse about HPV and cervical cancer, the young woman who becomes sexually active is positioned as one who has engaged (willingly or not) in risk-taking behavior. She has, in Perry's words, made a "wrong choice."

The risks associated with sex are positioned firmly within traditional, heterosexual gender role expectations, where accusations of promiscuity are an important mechanism for constraining young women's sexual activity. Such accusations point to the reemergence of a discourse of blame that is already at play with regard to cervical cancer and STIs more generally. Consider the response to Illinois state senator Debbie Halverson, the Democratic majority leader and sponsor of a mandate bill. The *New York Times* reports, "And in Illinois, a bill introduced by a legislator who had the virus the vaccine is intended to prevent prompted a conservative group's blog to speculate that she had been promiscuous."[114] The blogger at the heart of this controversy is Jill Stanek, who suggested in a post titled "Debbie Does . . . ??" (a title hinting at the title of a pornographic movie, *Debbie Does Dallas*) that Halvorson should offer an explanation for how she came to acquire the disease. Stanek asked Halvorson to "discuss the number of sex partners she has had throughout her lifetime" and explain to the public how, if she did not have multiple partners, it was possible for her to get the virus from her husband. Stanek also wrote that "if Halvorson contracted HPV through rape, she could discuss ways to avoid rape."[115] Stanek argued that Halvorson was advocating avoiding the consequences of risky behavior instead of avoiding the risky behavior itself. Positioned as a former risky young woman (now perhaps a risky woman), Halvorson is the recipient of a harsh judgment from the conservative press: by engaging in a risky act, she brought her illness—and its eventual remedy, a hysterectomy—upon herself.

Stanek's list of demands for Halvorson is useful in several ways for understanding the noncommercial discourse and its depiction of young women. First, if nothing else, Stanek demonstrates clearly that while sex may have been largely absent from commercial discourse—the Gardasil advertisements—it took the central role in noncommercial discourse as the primary risk young women face. Stanek literally defined sex as a risky behavior. Second, Stanek's indictment of Halvorson points to the fact that young women are always already both at risk and risky. Risky young women were once good girls, and the at-risk young women are always positioned as able to "fall off the path of virtue" and engage in risky behaviors. Such women are vulnerable in a number of ways: they are vulnerable to the consequences of the actions of others (often men, including future spouses and rapists) and to the consequences of their own actions. But although young women are held responsible for the risks they take when they engage in sex, they are not offered any positive mechanisms of control over their own sexuality. Stanek feels that young women should avoid sex; it is an act from which they need protection.

Commentators who promote abstinence-only education and those who opposed the mandate on other grounds emphasized the protection angle in their discussions of HPV and cervical cancer. Conservative activist Penna Dexter chastised parents who opted for the vaccine: "So, in order to protect their little girls, mothers are dragging them to the doctor for yet another shot, hoping to save them from certain decisions they might make someday about their sexuality, or from the pasts of their future sexual partners. It's a shame, but in America, we often go after the 'quick fix.' It's a lot easier to give your daughter a vaccine against a sexually transmitted disease than to build into her, during those 'teachable moments' beginning in childhood, the knowledge that sex is for marriage. But, instead, our culture has left our daughters adrift, without an anchor."[116] Although some abstinence-only messages also emphasize an empowerment angle (suggesting that young women are being empowered to say no), more often they resort to a paternalistic mode of protection in which the at-risk/risky young woman, unable to make sexual decisions for herself, is taught that sex before marriage is both physically and morally risky. For Dexter, protection occurs through knowledge and the hope that "young women whose morals are grounded in their faith have the tools to remain pure in an increasingly impure world."[117] Dexter's statements are just one example of a striking aspect of the paternalist narrative about HPV and cervical cancer: the young woman's utter lack of empowerment regarding sex. I move in the next section to an analysis of the young woman's means of empowerment and her full transformation into a vulnerable empowered woman in the second advertising campaign for Gardasil.

Empowering the At-Risk/Risky Young Woman: Gardasil's Second Campaign

By ceding discussions of sex to noncommercial public discourse and prompting a focus on the bodies and lives of privileged young women, Merck in effect helped create the very controversy it was trying to avoid. By mid-2007, Merck was attempting to diffuse the controversy. It retreated from public debates about the mandate, including withdrawing its financial support of Women in Government, in an effort to ease concerns about the influence of "Big Pharma" on public policy. In response to the outcry about young women and sex, Merck officials made statements about the vaccine's importance for preventing cervical cancer. Early in the development of the controversy, Dr. Richard M. Haupt, director for medical affairs in Merck's vaccine division, explained, "Our goal is to prevent cervical cancer."[118] In public statements Merck stayed true to an important aspect of the Gardasil girl narrative: Gardasil was a vaccine for cervical cancer. Merck did not engage in more explicit discussions of sex, sexuality, or even the nature of HPV as a sexually transmitted infection. However, the company launched a new campaign for Gardasil in 2008: the "I Chose" campaign.

The "I Chose" campaign is best interpreted as an accommodation to the outcry over the Gardasil mandates and the issue of young women's sexuality. It continued to use the slogan "One Less," but always with a specific "I Chose" statement such as "I chose to get vaccinated because I'll do everything I can to help protect myself from cervical cancer."[119] In many ways, the new "I

Chose" advertisements upped the postfeminist ante in the advertisements by more explicitly giving the power to choose to women (or at least some women). However, the "I Chose" advertisements also emphasized new aspects of the Gardasil girl identity that signaled the Gardasil girl's kinship with the young woman of noncommercial public discourse. In the "One Less" advertisements, the young women who give voice to the One Less mantra ("I want to be one less") are on the verge of full womanhood and full independence. Their bodies are ambiguously aged, and they are engaged in activities outside the home. These bodies are replaced in the "I Chose" campaign with bodies of younger girls in close contact with their mothers, often in domestic settings, and with bodies of adult women (also in domestic settings) who are clearly past their teenage years. In response to the growing furor over Gardasil mandates, the "I Chose" campaign returns the powerful (perhaps dangerous) adolescent bodies of the "One Less" campaign to their more proper, traditional, setting: home. The underlying message about the vaccine remains intact—the vaccine is necessary because it helps prevent cancer—but the "I Chose" commercials engage in a domestication of the Gardasil girl that brings her fully in alignment with the sexual politics behind the construction of the young woman. Even though Merck continued to avoid discussions of sex and sexuality, the problematic implications of women's sexuality as constructed in noncommercial discourse (sex is risky and young women must be protected from sex) haunt the depictions of women in "I Chose" campaign.

Of the three "I Chose" commercials I analyze, one was focused entirely on adult women. The women who speak are at least in their late teenage years (they are depicted as working professionals or college students). The women of this advertisement are the more adult embodiment of Gardasil girl. Unlike the adolescents of "One Less," who voice their desires ("I want to be one less"), the women of the adult commercial can directly and explicitly claim their empowerment through choice. The first two women in the commercial begin statements with "I chose to get vaccinated . . ."[120] Eight women are featured in the adult advertisement: four white women, three African American women, and one Asian woman. Despite their racial/ethnic diversity, they are uniform in both their middle-class status (one African American woman, for example, sits on a white couch with floral pillows, sipping a mug of coffee or tea and working on her laptop) and their location: all of the women are depicted in a domestic setting. Only two are not specifically in living rooms. Both are white women; one is sitting in a home studio overlooking a garden (she is painting), and a second is sitting in what appears to be a dorm room. As the womanly embodiment of the construct of the young woman, the women in this advertisement are not yet married and they do not have children, but they are in the position to be thinking about sexual activity. Indeed, as they note frequently, Gardasil does not just protect against cervical cancer, it also protects against "other HPV diseases."

The two other nationally aired commercials for the "I Chose" campaign featured mother/daughter pairs (for ease of reference, I discuss these commercials as "Pairs One" and "Pairs Two"). "Pairs One" returns young women to the outdoors, but only in the company of their mothers. Significantly, many of these adolescents do not look that different from those in the original "One Less" advertisements. The first mother/daughter pair is preparing to surf, and the daughter is a well-developed blonde who looks to be about fifteen years old. Placed in a different context, in a different advertisement, the young woman could easily be interpreted by audiences as a highly sexualized figure. The adolescent is accompanied by her mother (also in a wetsuit), who says, "Every day about thirty women in the U.S. learn they have cervical cancer. That's why I chose to get my daughter vaccinated."[121] With her mother standing next to her and making medical decisions for her, the potential sexuality of the young woman in the wetsuit is effectively reduced. Of the five mother/daughter pairs in this advertisement, three include daughters who are possibly pre-pubescent and thus culturally inappropriate objects of sexual attention. The youngest is an African American daughter who is in a swimming competition (her mother appears to be the coach). Her mother speaks directly to the youth of her daughter: "I chose to get my daughter vaccinated because the CDC recommends that girls her age get vaccinated."[122] These three individuals are bookended by the mother/daughter surfing pair and a Latina mother/daughter pair in which the daughter is wearing an elegant dress and high-heeled shoes and is receiving a necklace from her mother. They are in the living room of a house. This final scene can easily be interpreted as a moment from a quinceañera celebration, mimicking the multicultural, postracial approach of the "One Less" campaign and offering a specific age for the adolescent (she is turning fifteen). As with the young woman in the wetsuit, the young woman celebrating her quinceañera is beautiful and, in this case, dressed to the nines. Her mother's presence, however, signals her protected status and reduces (although not completely erases) the young woman's status as a sexual subject. The mixed settings (both home and away from home) of this advertisement disappear entirely in "Pairs Two," which offers only scenarios in domestic settings.[123] Further, within the home many of the pairs in the second advertisement are engaged in feminized activities. The first pair (white) is sitting on a couch (the daughter is holding a skateboard) in a living room; the second pair (African American) is in a kitchen, with the mother braiding her daughter's hair; the third pair (white) is sitting at a dining room table, with the mother painting her daughter's nails; the fourth pair (white) is in a kitchen talking; the fifth pair (white) is at a kitchen table playing checkers; and the sixth group (white, a mother with two daughters, or a daughter with a friend) is in the kitchen baking.

Combined, the "I Chose" commercials successfully domesticate the formerly autonomous Gardasil girl. In the second campaign, she is alone only when she is clearly an adult; until then, even as an older teenager, she is with her mother. The domestication of the Gardasil girl points to her sisterhood with the good young woman of public discourse. By domesticating the Gardasil girl and constraining her sexuality until she is clearly an adult, Merck's second advertising campaign engages in the same sexual politics as the noncommercial discourse. While the "I Chose" campaign still does not identify HPV as a sexually transmitted infection (and thus does not discuss sex openly), it protects young women from the risk of sex by placing her (in her pre-adolescent and adolescent years) in the care of her mother (often in a domestic location) and by confining her (as an adult) to domestic spaces (dormitory rooms, home offices, living rooms). Sex in this sense haunts the "I Chose" commercials to the extent that through Merck's depictions of the domesticated young girls, adolescents, and adult young women, the distinction between the Gardasil girl and the young woman disappears. Together, the noncommercial discourse about the young woman and the newly domesticated Gardasil girl of the "I Chose" campaign offer the public a depiction of heterosexual womanhood with one driving telos: reproduction.

After the young woman becomes the central character in both commercial and noncommercial discourse, her means of empowerment is clear, if also limited and problematic. Although she continues to be disempowered in relation to sex, the young woman in the "I Chose" campaign can choose to be vaccinated. This choice, however, is given only to women who are adults or are nearing adulthood. In the "I Chose" commercial featuring adult women, the women state their choice to be vaccinated: "I chose to get vaccinated when my doctor told me that HPV can affect women my age and how Gardasil can help protect me."[124] The adult commercial ends with the words "Choose to get vaccinated" appearing on the screen and a voiceover announcing, "You have the power to choose. Ask your doctor about Gardasil." But this power to choose is not given to most of the adolescents in the mother/daughter pair commercials. In "Pairs One," for example, four mothers offer statements that include the words "I chose to get my daughter vaccinated" followed by why they made the choice.[125] The one daughter who speaks gives some medical information but does not even give voice to a desire to be "one less." In "Pairs Two," mothers are again featured as choosing the vaccination for their daughters. The first mother states, "I chose to get my daughter vaccinated because I want her to be one less woman affected by cervical cancer."[126] The "I Chose" campaign carefully delineates between younger girls who need to have others make choices for them and adults who can choose on their own and thus preserves the discourse of protection for the youngest of girls. As they grow, however, these young girls gain knowledge of the vaccine, and some gain the power to speak about that knowledge. For example, at the beginning of "Pairs One," a mother/daughter pair is getting ready to surf. The mother opens the commercial by explaining her reasons for vaccinating her daughter. The commercial then introduces three new mother/daughter pairs, each with their own message, and returns about midway through to the adolescent surfer daughter, who explains, "Gardasil does not treat cervical cancer or other HPV diseases." This daughter is given a voice and knowledge about the vaccine. With her mother's assistance, she can move toward enacting the postfeminist mechanism of empowerment: choosing the vaccine. The ending of "Pairs Two" captures the balance between protection and empowerment perfectly. As the voiceover declares "Gardasil. You have the power to choose. Ask your daughter's doctor about Gardasil," the words "Choose to get vaccinated" appear on the screen.[127] These messages speak to both the young woman ("Choose to get vaccinated") and her mother ("Ask your daughter's doctor about Gardasil").

Paternalism, Postfeminism, and Why a Feminist Perspective on Women's Health Matters

In combination, the commercial and noncommercial discourses about the HPV vaccine offer a perfect snapshot of the empowerment/protection paradox at work in public discourse about HPV and cervical cancer. The adolescents and young adults in the Gardasil commercials speak of their desire to be one less woman with cervical cancer and of the choices they have made to fulfill that desire. In noncommercial discourse, only a very few young women speak, and they speak, like Amanda Vail and Heather Burcham, who supported Perry's executive order, only after they have contracted the disease. The rest of the young women are silenced, and adults—parents, politicians, bloggers, doctors, researchers, and journalists—skirmish over the best way to protect them. What can we make of the identity of the at-risk/risky young woman who, even though she is empowered to desire and choose certain medical treatments, is silenced about sexuality? How should we understand a young woman who is firmly situated in biomedicine and remains tethered to a good/bad girl dichotomy in which nearly any sexual behavior she is involved in (whether it is an action done to her or an action she chooses) is her responsibility? The at-risk/risky young woman is, I would suggest, an identity that captures the often hidden threat of postfeminism.

One of the difficulties in critiquing postfeminist culture is that it is so incessantly positive, particularly in terms of the cultural phenomenon of girl power. Girls can do anything: they can be rock stars, presidents, tomboys and sex kittens. And in most media representations of girl power, they can do and be many of these things without consequences. Girls are empowered. But a critical look at these messages of girl power leads us back to my concern with the brand of empowerment postfeminism offers: girls, young women, and adult women are offered empowerment mainly through consumption, and this type of empowerment serves to further entrench them within traditional gender roles.

I titled this chapter "The Postfeminist Concession," and it is worth taking a moment to think about what exactly postfeminism kept and what it conceded. What postfeminist discourse maintained was a version of women's empowerment in the medical sphere. This mode of empowerment is limited by age (even older adolescents need parental approval) and it continues the neoliberal model of empowerment through choice and consumption and the largely unquestioning nature of that consumption. The ability to vaccinate young individuals, both girls and boys, against HPV and thus avoid (or at the very least decrease the risk of) at least three different kinds of cancer (cervical, anal, and penile) as well as genital warts is precisely the type of "hope technology" that the era of biomedicalization offers the public.[128] However, in commercial and noncommercial public discourse the act of choosing the vaccine is joined by a forgetting of the fact that access to medical choice is unequal (in this case, the only individuals who can choose are privileged), a near-complete neglect of the controversies about the efficacy and safety of the vaccine, and a reliance on traditional gender roles for young women.[129] Indeed, what postfeminism conceded was the pretense of women's sexual agency. This was replaced by a more forthright and explicitly conservative and patriarchal discussion that took place entirely within the norms of the heterosexual matrix. With this concession in mind, the at-risk/risky young woman is the embodiment of postfeminism's threat to women: the ease with which postfeminism can incorporate or be incorporated into explicitly patriarchal understandings of womanhood.

Paula Treichler's idea of the burdens of history regarding women and STIs is useful in understanding the dynamics of public discourse about HPV and cervical cancer. Young women simply cannot escape the stigma of STIs, and, because HPV was solidified as a women's health issue in the early years of the vaccine, even the addition of men into the discourse of HPV is unlikely to disrupt the overall messages about sex and sexuality: sex is dangerous, young women are morally virtuous only if they are sexually pure, and although they can hope to decrease their risk of cervical cancer by using the vaccine (or even by having regular Pap smears), they remain at the mercy of their (risky) sexuality and the (dangerous) men around them.[130] On a broader scale, the identity constructed for young women—or those in the nine-to-twenty-six-year age range of the vaccine—also has ramifications for older adult women, in part because of the reproductive function of the young woman identity. Where does the adult woman who does not have children or the adult woman who is not fully engaged in the heterosexual matrix belong? The short answer: at the edge of discourse, invisible, next to the equally invisible ranks of poor women and women of color.

An emphasis on women's reproduction has been a common theme of this book. This emphasis points to one of the larger dangers of postfeminist discourse about women's health, and this danger is particularly well displayed in the case study about cervical cancer. Despite its messages of empowerment for women and girls of all ages, postfeminism is disempowering in some of the arenas where feminists have worked so hard to gain empowerment: women's role in the home, familial and sexual relationships, and reproduction. Instead, postfeminism offers women consumption as their main means of empowerment—a distinctly neoliberal option.

On the one hand, this mode of empowerment is precisely what social theorist Nikolas Rose offers some support for when he notes that in the twenty-first century we are in the midst of a new politics of life in which biology is no longer destiny.[131] Through choices—about which drugs to consume, which treatments to pursue, which doctors to call upon—we participate in the crafting of ourselves. On the other hand, empowerment through which medical services we choose can be problematic because of the larger discursive and lived contexts in which such choices take shape. For example, the choice of whether or not to get the HPV vaccine is tied directly to a postfeminist understanding of womanhood in public discourse and seems to be the only mechanism of empowerment offered to women. Further, as consumers of the vaccine (or as consumers of prophylactic mastectomies or psychiatric pharmaceuticals), women are not represented as engaging critically with biomedicine. In public discourse, women do not ask questions about the safety and efficacy of medical treatments or why research has focused on some treatments over others. When they are incorporated into postfeminist discourse, neoliberal ideas of choice support women's unquestioning engagement with biomedicine, an engagement that aligns with a revitalization of some of the oldest and most traditional gender roles for women: the obedient and virtuous daughter who becomes an obedient and fertile wife.

Chapter 5

Feminist Women's Health Activism in the Twenty-first Century

In this chapter, I offer one possible vision for a feminist women's health politics in the twenty-first century that attempts to answer some of the substantial problems with the postfeminist narratives about women's health that circulate in mainstream public discourse. In the conclusion of their 1999 edited volume *Revisioning Women, Health and Healing,* Virginia Olesen and Adele Clarke refuse to support a specific agenda for feminist health activists, instead suggesting that a more pragmatic move is to "embrace agendas of problematizing, reconceptualizing, retheorizing, and revisioning any and all topics within women, health, and healing, especially those that derive from and are found in distinctively cultural arenas that limit women's potentials and produce inequities and injustices."[1] Like Olesen and Clarke, I am hesitant to offer support to only one feminist agenda or feminist vision of women's health. Thus, what I offer in this chapter should be understood as one vision, one specific way of reconceptualizing a feminist approach to women's health. I begin by offering a discussion of the context for women's health activism today, including a final critique of the core themes of postfeminist narratives about women's health and the postfeminist identities offered to women. I then turn to examples of contemporary feminist activism that illuminate the three potential areas of focus for a feminist vision of women's health. I conclude by arguing that the lack of a single agenda for feminist health activists should be embraced, not feared, as such diversity in agendas has the potential to create a multiplicity of new public narratives that can increase the variety of subjectivities offered to women.

The New Context of Women's Health Activism

In May 2010, the birth control pill celebrated its fiftieth anniversary. In May 1960, the FDA approved Enovid, an estrogen/progestin pill created by Searle for the American market specifically for use as contraception. A *New York Times* article, titled "It Started More Than a Revolution," offers one take on the Pill's importance: it brought about a "kind of reformation" in terms of drug regulation. Reporter Gardiner Harris describes how the FDA had been fitfully moving toward stricter regulations of pharmaceuticals in the early 1960s, in part because of the thalidomide crisis in Europe (the drug had never been approved in the United States). With the Pill's growing popularity (within four years of approval, over four million women had used it) came evidence that it was not entirely safe; reports of women dying because of blood clots were available by 1961. In 1965, the FDA established its first permanent advisory panel to track the Pill's safety. In addition, the FDA took the extraordinary step of communicating directly with patients through prescription inserts. The FDA had been locked in a struggle with the powerful American Medical Association about who could talk to patients for many years. Gardiner explains the situation in 1970: "The challenge of communicating these risks to patients while still supporting the product's use bedeviled top agency officials." Because doctors refused to give patients informational material about the Pill provided by the FDA (arguing that the agency was intruding on doctor-patient relationships), the FDA finally mandated in 1978 that the handouts be given to women when they picked up their prescriptions. In the narrative constructed in Gardiner's article, Peter Barton Hutt, a former FDA lawyer, offers this final statement: "The pill was a landmark in the field of drug regulation. This is the drug that started it all."[2]

What is remarkable about the narrative about the safety regulations put in place after the Pill entered the U.S. market is how the Pill itself becomes the instigator for change. Almost entirely missing are the women's health activists who worked tirelessly to bring the Pill's dangers to the attention of both the FDA and Congress. In the *Times* article, such activists receive one line: "Protests by women's groups and hearings on Capitol Hill made clear that despite the agency's attempts, many women said they took the pill without being fully informed of its risks."[3] Not only does this statement reduce the FDA's responsibility (the tone suggests that it was doing its best), but it also hints at women's responsibility: Why would they take a pill without being fully informed first? An article in *Ms.* by Elizabeth Kissling, also published in May 2010, countered this narrative. Its title was "How the Pill Gave Birth to the Women's Health

Movement."[4] Unlike the story in the *Times*, the feminist recounting of the Pill remembers the women's health movement and suggests that women's health activists changed the shape of the FDA regulatory process by insisting upon greater safety regulations and that extensive information be given to patients. The 1970 congressional hearings on the Pill that were prompted in part by the publication in 1969 of Barbara Seaman's scathing critique of the pill, its safety, and the medical industry's cover-up, *The Doctor's Case Against the Pill*, are pivotal in the feminist recounting. Kissling explains how activists such as Barbara Seaman and Alice Koffman disrupted the hearings, shouting a series of questions to senators who refused to allow them to testify officially: "Why weren't we told about side effects? Why aren't any women testifying? What happened to the women in the Puerto Rico study? Why are you using women as guinea pigs?"[5]

The disruption of the hearings may have appeared unseemly, but it was effective. Seaman, Koffman, and the activists had the attention of the senators and more importantly, the media. Kissling explains the importance of the hearings: "The Nelson pill hearings eventually led to lower doses of estrogen in the pill (today's oral contraceptives are about 1/10th the strength of Enovid) and perhaps, more importantly, the introduction of patient package inserts, PPIs. The new FDA requirements resulted in the inclusion of printed information about risks, ingredients and side effects in pill packets, and eventually in all pharmaceuticals."[6]

These two articles—published within a few days of each other—demonstrate the erasure of the women's health movement in mainstream public discourse. Where the feminist writer of *Ms.* situates the FDA's new regulations as a response to growing pressure by women's health activists, the *Times* situates the regulations as part of a larger shift by the FDA, spurred on by Congress, the haunting stories about thalidomide, and reports of the Pill's dangers and problems, to more carefully consider issues regarding drug safety and efficacy. This erasure is only a symptom of a larger phenomenon. Feminism does not need to be remembered in public discourse because postfeminism claims that feminism has achieved its goal of equality for women. In contemporary public discourse about women's health, equality is presented as equal representation in medical studies, the increased public visibility of women's health, and the ever-increasing choices women can make about their health. While public discourse about women's health issues points to the success of the women's health movement, the postfeminist nature of that discourse suggests the need to revisit what feminist health activism can look like—and accomplish—in the twenty-first century.

Neoliberalism, Postfeminism, and the U.S. Healthcare System

When feminist health activists emerged on the scene in the late 1960s and early 1970s, women interfaced with a very different health system than they do now. Reflecting on this period, public health scholars Sheryl Burt Ruzek and Julie Becker write, "The assumption was simply that physicians were the experts and women were to do as instructed."[7] Women discussed their health problems privately with their physicians in an inhospitable medical environment. The layperson's access to medical information was restricted. Very little research was being done on women's health issues, and women were routinely excluded in clinical trials. Women were also excluded as practitioners; in the early part of the twentieth century and through the mid-1960s, women constituted only about 5 percent of medical students.[8] In a medical environment that opposed women's access to knowledge of and control over their own bodies, the successes of the women's health movement's activists are striking; the new FDA regulations about the birth control pill is but one of many examples. Women's health movement activists won battles in almost every arena, including reproductive rights and breast cancer awareness and treatment. Furthermore, women's health activists demanded medical accountability in situations where medical treatments offered to women were found to be dangerous. As just one example, the feminist press covered the emerging story of diethylstilbestrol (DES) in the early 1970s. DES, a form of estrogen, was given to approximately three million pregnant women in the United States between 1945 and 1970 to prevent miscarriages and was linked by the late 1960s to a deadly form of uterine cancer in the daughters of women who had taken the drug. The American Medical Association recommended that doctors who used DES in their practice should warn their patients, but most doctors failed to comply. In response, feminist activists formed two groups, the Coalition for the Medical Rights of Women and DES Action, to alert DES daughters and sons of health problems associated with DES. Perhaps the most striking success of the women's health movement was the fact that it made women's health issues publicly visible, a visibility that increased not just public awareness of women's health but also influenced medical research agendas. Sociologist Steven Epstein suggests that although "different political 'lines' within feminism had different effects," all contributed to the increasing attention paid to research on women's health.[9] This increase in visibility was accompanied by an increase in biotechnology but also by a new (and potentially problematic) understanding of the meaning of difference in the health arena. The current paradigm of inclusion and difference has prompted the widespread recognition that "sometimes the pursuit of genuine social equality requires policies that do not treat everyone the same," but at the same time this paradigm has the potential to reify the very differences (for example, sex difference) that many feminist health activists were attempting to break down.[10] Furthermore, the visibility of women's health is now intimately tied to profit-making medical corporations. Neoliberal marketing strategies have effectively blurred the line between medical research and marketing of pharmaceutical drugs and illnesses.

Women's health issues, once in the shadows, are now ubiquitous, but they are framed through a postfeminist logic that promises women choices, most often in terms of what medical product they wish to consume. Ruzek and Becker, reflecting on this change, suggest that part of the new dynamic is the decreasing influence of grassroots women's health organizations such as the National Women's Health Network (NWHN) that were founded by feminist women's health activists in the 1970s. The NWHN (founded by Barbara Seaman and colleagues soon after the hearings on the pill) is facing "declining support from both individuals and foundations as they compete with newer [professional, one-issue advocacy] organizations for members and resources."[11] Professional women's health organizations are evidence of the growing influence of neoliberalism on the politics of health. Simply stated, the emerging "equality politics" of neoliberalism emphasize global consumption and the upward redistribution of resources.[12] This is a form of equality that differs dramatically from what was envisioned by the social movements of the 1960s and 1970s. Movements like the women's liberation movement and the civil rights movement were diverse in terms of specific issues but did share one broad goal in common: downward redistribution. American Studies scholar Lisa Duggan explains: "In their hybrid, mongrel mixtures the overall emphasis that connected the progressive-left social movements was the pressure to level hierarchies and redistribute *down*—redistribute money, political power, cultural capital, pleasure, and freedom."[13] Professional organizations such as the Komen Foundation and the Ovarian Cancer National Alliance do important work, but while they speak for women, they are not necessarily feminist.[14] Ruzek and Becker point to one of the underlying problems with such organizations: they depend on and collaborate with the medical industry. They explain, "The women's health movement critique of biomedicine and the call for demedicalizing women's health care was reframed into a bipartisan agenda for equity" in access to federal funding and attention from the medical industry.[15] One of the legacies of women's health movement—the "deep skepticism toward the mainstream medical profession"—has not been incorporated into the messages or the stance of professional women's health organizations.[16] The absence of an overtly critical perspective of some professional women's health organizations is a significant part of the new health care landscape that promotes postfeminist, neoliberal messages about women's health.

The Problems of Postfeminist Women's Health Discourse

The case studies that make up this project have touched on a variety of topics—motherhood, sexuality, good womanhood—in addition to the health topics at hand. In this section, I offer a concise explanation for why the meanings that have been constructed for breast cancer, postpartum depression, and cervical cancer and the identities these discourses offer women—the cancer/risk-free woman, the risky mother, and the at-risk/risky young woman—are problematic from a feminist perspective. In addition to their common grounding in postfeminist and neoliberal discourses, what ties the case studies together is how these constructions reduce the complexity of women's lives to simplistic and limited identities. The narratives of women facing breast cancer, postpartum depression, and cervical cancer offer the public only a small portion of the broad range of women's experiences. Below, I discuss four specific issues—the focus on elite women, the reification of traditional gender roles, the affirmation of the power of biomedicine, and the depoliticization of women's health—that together demonstrate the potential dangers of a postfeminist vision of women's health.

Postfeminism and Privileged Women

In her discussion of postfeminism, Mary Douglas Vavrus explains that postfeminist ideology assumes "that white, heterosexual, middle-class women's issues can be generalized to all women, including those whose identities include none of these traits."[17] The elitism of postfeminism is apparent in contemporary mainstream representations of women's health. With very few exceptions, the women who make up the focus of public discourse about women's health are white, heterosexual, and middle to upper class. Constructed as vulnerable empowered women, they are firmly situated in a relationship with biomedicine as their bodies present vulnerabilities—framed as risks—that women must mitigate. Such public discourse about women's health does little to answer to the very real inequalities in access to health care and to health itself that exist for groups of women in the United States: women of different racial/ethnic backgrounds, of different sexualities, of different classes, and so forth. Postfeminist representations repeat one of the problems that the feminist women's health movement of the 1970s struggled to rectify in its own work: a focus on the lives of white, middle-class women.

The case of cervical cancer and the HPV vaccine is a particularly good example of the ramifications of focusing on elite women. The medical researchers who created the vaccine were aware of disparities in the incidence of and mortality from cervical cancer both nationally and globally. These disparities are directly connected to a variety of socioeconomic and cultural factors that make it difficult for women to have access to regular pap smears and follow-up treatment when necessary.[18] Yet a combination of factors—first the post-feminist Gardasil girl narrative in the advertisements for Gardasil and then the transformation of the Gardasil girl into a young woman in noncommercial discourse—worked to present an identity that limited concern about HPV and cervical cancer to the bodies and lives of privileged, postracial adolescents. The identities of at-risk/risky young women are premised on young women's sexual purity, and sexual purity is always already raced and classed in a specific way.

To be clear, I am not arguing that the vaccine should be mandated for all women indiscriminately or even that women should choose to have the vaccine; the newness of the vaccine and the lack of clarity about its long-term safety and efficacy should give feminist activists pause. What I am suggesting is that the narrowing of the discussion about HPV and cervical cancer on the postracial (read: white) figure of adolescent purity works to displace concern for women of color, poor women, and lesbian women in public discourse. As just one example of this displacement, when the U.S. Citizenship and Immigration Services mandated the HPV vaccine for green card applicants and immigrants applying for citizenship in July 2008, the ruling received little attention from the mainstream media. The new mandate was challenged by over one hundred progressive advocacy groups, who sent the clear message that "the singling out of immigrant women would not be tolerated."[19] Miriam Yeung and Amanda Allen critiqued the mandate because of its failure to recognize the real problems behind health disparities: "Reducing health disparities faced by immigrant women requires greatly expanded access to culturally competent medical services and effective measures to make health care more affordable. In addition, expanding access to and encouraging voluntary use of a vaccine like Gardasil among immigrant populations requires a combination of genuine, informed consent and efforts to increase the affordability for immigrant women of the vaccine."[20] Although progressive groups were successful in their challenge to this mandate (the requirement for the vaccine was dropped in 2010), my search for mainstream news coverage of the issue returned only a handful of sources.[21] Thus, not only are women who do not meet the postfeminist ideal largely invisible in public discourse, but feminist and progressive conversations about how to approach the issue of health disparities constructively are also effectively erased.

Postfeminism and Traditional Womanhood

Postfeminism promises women equality. However, the equality offered to women through postfeminist women's health discourse—namely, equality through neoliberal discourses of choice and self-discipline—is always undergirded by traditional gender roles. In public discourse about health and medicine, traditional gender roles appear to play a significant role in discussions of ways to stay healthy and why staying healthy should be important. Public discourse about postpartum depression continues to exist in dialogue with a larger discourse about good mothering, in this case risky mothering. Similarly, the traditional role of the sexually pure young woman who will soon be a wife and mother emerges as pivotal in public discussions of HPV and cervical cancer.

The case study of breast cancer, however, perhaps offers us the most unique way that traditional understandings of womanhood are used to suggest how the cancer/risk-free woman should act in the face of the risks posed by the BRCA genetic mutation. Prophylactic mastectomies are represented as a compulsory choice for women with the BRCA genetic mutation, and although this happens in part through an emphasis on the horrors of the disease, one of the reasons for having a prophylactic mastectomy is clear: to ensure women's ability to have a family (that is, to become a wife and mother) in the future. For women who already have a family, the "how" of staying healthy—again, the prophylactic mastectomy—is supported in these representations by much the same reasoning: prophylactic mastectomies ensure a woman's continued ability to perform her role as wife and mother. When I wrote the chapter on prophylactic mastectomies, Christina Applegate and Jessica Queller were represented as facing very loudly ticking biological clocks. Queller was the most insistent upon her desire to become a mother, and as of mid-2009, she had successfully become pregnant through artificial insemination. In 2011, Applegate gave birth to a baby girl, a "miracle" according to *People* magazine.[22] In the media, these pregnancies are presented as the end points of long, and successful, journeys to have a family. Renée Montagne's introduction of Jessica Queller implicitly points to the journey metaphor: "When we spoke to her, she had not yet had her ovaries removed, the only way to guarantee that she won't get ovarian cancer. That's because she wanted to have a baby and made the decision to try and have one on her own. . . . And I should say congratulations, because you are, indeed, pregnant."[23] The coverage of Applegate is similar; one article called the news of her pregnancy "joyful" and counted the months until Applegate's "little family will be complete."[24] Taken together, the three case studies in this book leave little doubt about how important the role of motherhood is constructed to be in the lives of postfeminist vulnerable empowered women.

Postfeminism and Biomedicine

At the beginning of the case study of postpartum depression, I outlined the efforts of feminist psychologists and postpartum self-help groups to recognize and emphasize the need for attention to be paid to the social and structural contexts of mothering and to at the same time advocate for proper diagnosis and treatment of women with postpartum disorders. This case study offers perhaps the clearest example of the medicalization of women's lives, on at least two levels. The identity of the risky mother normalizes postpartum depression by accepting the medicalized understanding of postpartum depression. The privileged women at the center of the narrative of risky motherhood are understood to be good mothers who can be depressed. Depression has a clear source (hormones that influence neurotransmitters) and a clear treatment (antidepressants). Although the normalization of postpartum depression alleviates some of the stigma associated with depression (and even some of the stigma associated with psychosis, as long as the child is not harmed), it does little to attempt to understand women's lives, bodies, and experiences with explanations that are not medical. The process of medicalization is complete for the risky mother when her role as a mother is forever tied to the role of patient: she is surveilled by doctors, friends, family members, husband, and herself.

The medicalization of postpartum depression is only one way postfeminist depictions of women's health work in concert with the medical industry. The power of biomedicine is upheld through the methods of empowerment offered to the vulnerable empowered woman. Each time a risk is understood, the vulnerable empowered woman must act, and her actions are directed toward medical solutions. The risky mother takes pharmaceutical medications and is at times is hospitalized in order to continue functioning as a good mother. The cancer/risk-free woman of the prophylactic mastectomy narrative undergoes substantial, radical surgery to avoid cancer and continues to rely upon the medical establishment to help her recraft her body. The at-risk/risky young woman of the cervical cancer discourse is disempowered in relation to her body and her sexuality, but when she is old enough, she is empowered to desire and then choose to be vaccinated. Relying upon biomedicine for their health, these vulnerable empowered women are empowered make choices that imply—and indeed require—their unquestioning trust in the medical system. Substantial critiques of the path of breast cancer research, the efficacy of the Gardasil vaccine, or the belief that hormones alone cause postpartum depression disappear. The vulnerable woman's empowerment depends on her intimate and long-term relationship with biomedicine. To be clear, biomedical understandings of our bodies and selves can be beneficial. Sociologist Nikolas Rose suggests, for example, that such understandings allow us to experience ourselves in a new way and offer new possibilities for living.[25] However, as represented through the identity of the vulnerable empowered woman, the woman with postpartum depression, breast cancer, or cervical cancer has few options for empowerment outside the realm of biomedicine, and within that realm she is only rarely depicted as questioning or critiquing the very services she consumes.

Postfeminism and the Depoliticization of Women's Health

In a letter written to the National Women's Health Network days after the attacks on the World Trade Center in 2001 and in response to the network's mailer attacking President George W. Bush's record on women's health issues, Rosemary Hertz expressed her dismay with NWHN's tactics. She wrote, "Your organization is supposed to be a HEALTH ORGANIZATION and not a POLITICAL ORGANIZATION."[26] In this case, the writer's outrage with the NWHN is directly linked to the historical moment: it was politically impossible to attack Bush in the days after the 9/11 attacks. However, Hertz was also pointing to a larger issue: for her, the subject of health was not political. The depoliticization of women's health in postfeminist women's health discourse occurs through the crafting of meanings for women's health issues and identities for women. Breast cancer, for example, is constructed as an individual problem—a genetic problem—with a medical solution that individuals choose. In the prophylactic mastectomy narrative, the cancer/risk-free woman enacts this definition: she recognizes her genetic vulnerability and resolves it by having surgery. The consequences of focusing on individual women in public discourse (even when they are presented as a group in professional organizations) include a sustained ignorance about the (potential) environmental causes of breast cancer because of an insistence on looking to individuals and genetics for the cause. In other words, the depoliticization of breast cancer, the individualization of breast cancer, affects research agendas.

I would suggest that the depoliticization of women's health is most evident in what might seem like the most politicized of case studies: that of cervical cancer and the Gardasil vaccine. Politics were clearly a part of the HPV vaccine controversy and the narrative about the at-risk/risky young woman. Indeed, the politics of sex were all too clear; the discourse about young women and sexuality that framed sex as an immoral activity for women was frequently deployed by both supporters and detractors of the vaccination mandates. Nevertheless, this discourse (even in its highly politicized form) followed the same road that had been paved by the breast cancer and postpartum depression narratives: cancer and sexually transmitted infections were the problems of individual young women. Young women were seen as individually responsible for avoiding HPV by avoiding sex. They were given the option, in the Gardasil advertisements, to protect themselves through the vaccine. One aspect of the depoliticization of women's health is the absence of collective grassroots action, and here I do not mean action such as the lobbying done by many professional/neoliberal women's health groups. There was professionalized collective action—by groups such as Focus on the Family—to squash most of the mandates across the country. And there was action by the Merck-supported advocacy group Women in Government to continue sponsoring mandate legislation. But collective action by women—adolescents, young adults, and adults—disappeared almost entirely. Instead, the at-risk/risky young woman is empowered in much the same way as the risky mother and the cancer/risk-free woman: she is told to focus on herself, her risks, and her responsibilities to avoid and/or mitigate those risks. In this narrative, self-discipline has replaced political action. The choices public discourse offers to the vulnerable empowered woman are neoliberal choices: consumption and surveillance.[27]

The Feminist Counter to the Postfeminist Public:
Envisioning a New Feminist Health Politics

The dominant narratives about women's health reflect a broader social shift toward neoliberalism and postfeminism. These narratives exist in what I have discussed as mainstream public discourse: they are widely available through the nightly news, national newspapers, popular blogs, and best-selling books. But although postfeminist narratives about women's health are the most visible, they are not the *only* narratives available. As Phaedra Pezzullo argues in her discussion of public performances that critique National Breast Cancer Awareness Month (NBCAM), feminist activists working on women's health form a "counter-public" to the dominant discourses of women's health in the public sphere.[28] Work by feminist activists on the edge of mainstream discourse is important, as it always holds the potential to disrupt the dominant postfeminist hegemony. Pezzullo's study, for example, focused on how breast cancer activists (often members of Breast Cancer Action) use a variety of strategies to reframe, or rethink, the typical breast cancer survivor narrative. The performances of the Toxic Links Coalition's (TLC) "Stop Cancer Where it Starts" tours disrupt the normative discursive logics of NBCAM by developing new understandings of breast cancer.[29] The pink ribbon, for example, becomes a symbolic noose on the posters of activists, pointing to the ribbon's potential to gag and literally silence voices of dissent in the breast cancer community.

Women's health activists such as those working with TLC and BCA have created new strategies of disruption and new forms of feminist knowledge that meet the challenges of corporatized, neoliberal health care. Thus, the "Stop Cancer Where it Starts" tour asks participants to consider how corporations that often promise to be working with or for women to fight breast cancer are actually part of a larger cancer industrial complex that makes profits from and at times even causes cancer. Tactics such as these make up one aspect of a larger and dynamic new feminist vision of women's health. According to Nikolas Rose, "Many years ago now, when feminists proclaimed 'our bodies, ourselves,' they envisaged a very different form of politics, one in which the body was a natural object, which we must rescue from its alienated state, retrieve from the grasp of experts, which we can and should each know and tend for ourselves. . . . Now our bodies form the basis of many related but different projects in ways that could not have been anticipated in the critiques of medical authority in the 1960s and 1970s. . . . In this sense, our bodies have become ourselves, become central to our expectations, hopes, our individual and collective identities, and our biological responsibilities in this emergent form of life."[30] A new feminist health politics must be attuned to the differences between the eras of medicalization and biomedicalization and must (as Rose describes) be able to speak to the neoliberal reconsideration of the politics of life in which our bodies have become ourselves. To this end, the core themes of the women's health movement—attention to the politics of knowledge, self-determination, and contextualization—may play radically different roles (or no role at all) in a new feminist health politics. As just one example, the feminist emphasis on bodily self-determination (the right to bodily ownership) that was the focus of much of the abortion rights arguments in the women's health movement may not be as successful in a context in which the fetal body is also perceived to have rights (and can be manipulated and operated on with the same focus on bodily perfection as for adult bodies) and women are depicted as engaging in a series of freely made choices (to have sex or not, to use birth control or not) that position them as morally responsible for any pregnancy. In the next three sections, I delineate possible areas of focus for a new feminist health politics. I am primarily concerned with areas in which a new feminist health politics can provide an answer to or challenge some of the problems of postfeminist public discourse about women's health, recognizing of course that a new feminist health politics must also be responsive to the structural and institutional dynamics of biomedicine.

The Promise of Activism

In a context of new biotechnologies such as genetic testing and an increasing focus on women's ability (indeed, any person's ability) to manage individual risk by changing or modifying their bodies and lives for a better future, health becomes understood as the responsibility of individuals. Critics of biomedicalization and larger neoliberal risk discourse, including myself, are concerned with the ways such individualization often neglects or displaces concern about larger issues that may include the individual but move beyond the individual. Laura Mamo describes this phenomenon in terms of fertility: "Ideals of ownership and individualism punctuate reproductive practices and services as reproduction becomes another do-it-yourself project enabling us to transform our selves, identities, and social lives through consumption."[31] An understanding of reproduction as "do-it-yourself" self-transformation leaves untouched broader social and economic concerns, including issues of access to reproductive technologies and the possible privileging of heterosexuality (and/or a nuclear family ideal). Focusing on the individual's ability to manage the self works in many cases to reduce our vision of health to what an individual can do, what the individual is responsible for, and what the effect on the individual is of any given service or treatment.

In contrast to the strong critiques of the process of individualization, a different perspective on the focus of the self and new biotechnologies suggests that the biomedical era does not individualize at all; rather, such new technologies can be understood as making connections between individuals. Regarding genetics, Rose notes that "information that I may find out about my genetic complement traces new connections and imposes new obligations, between myself, my parents, relatives, brothers, sisters and my children, including those born through the donation of my sperm."[32] Instead of a rise of individualism, we might use the focus on genetics and individual risk factors to prompt a new form of sociality. Using Paul Rabinow's term "biosociality," Rose explains that "biosocial communities, often geographically dispersed, sometimes virtual, are brought into existence around a shared condition; they actively strive for research, for funds, for support, for therapies, for 'their disease.'"[33] Biosocial communities often focus on the work of awareness and fund-raising: in relation to their new somatic identities, individuals lobby politicians, work for more funded research, and in general enact "biological citizenship by demanding their rights for attention to their particular disorder."[34] In addition, biosocial communities can take up the work of living with a disease. Focusing on online communities of individuals with Huntington's disease, Carlos Novas suggests that individuals are not content with being passive subjects of medicogenetic knowledge and instead become "lay experts" who develop and share knowledge online.[35] Individuals within the community also engage in creating "life strategies" formulated in a complex ethical field that attempt to answer the question of how one should conduct one's life.[36] Biosocial communities are the most recent iteration of disease-related sociality, and today groups that are formed specifically around a genetic identity work for research, awareness, and fund-raising in ways that are many times (but not always) parallel to other health advocacy and/or support organizations.[37] For example, the group FORCE (Facing Our Risk of Cancer Empowered) is a biosocial community developed by and for women with the BRCA genetic mutation. In the United States, FORCE coexists with dozens of other breast cancer organizations, including other grassroots organizations and professional health advocacy groups.

If one critique of the process of individualization is its lack of a wider focus on social, economic, and even environmental issues, we could levy a similar critique at some of the work of the many different types of health advocacy and/or support organizations that now work on behalf of individuals with certain diseases, from biosocial communities to organizations such as Komen for the Cure. Specifically, what is often missing from such organizations is a notion of activism that moves beyond raising awareness about a disease, raising funds for medical research, and the creation and communication of lay/expert knowledge about how to live a successful life with certain genetic attributes and/or risk factors. To be clear, these are all significant actions, and groups that form around certain diseases have no doubt moved their issues into the spotlight, garnering more attention and more research funding. However, one potential area of focus for a new feminist health politics could be to bring a different type of activist orientation to health advocacy and/or support organizations or to create organizations with an explicitly activist orientation.

The grassroots organization Breast Cancer Action recounts its beginnings by focusing on one individual—Elenore Pred—and her anger regarding the lack of treatment options and information about metastatic breast cancer. BCA's website recounts, "In 1990, after years of encountering government agencies and organizations that provided inadequate and superficial information rather than scientific evidence about breast cancer, Elenore Pred grew angry. She shared her anger with other women who had metastatic breast cancer. Together they formed Breast Cancer Action (BCA), now a national organization at the forefront of the breast cancer activist movement."[38] One interpretation of the history of BCA is that Pred's experience as a biological citizen, one who could use the language of biology to describe her identity and her body with breast cancer as well as one who could take a dynamic interest in enhancing her own scientific literacy, enabled her to reach out and form an activist collective around the issue of breast cancer.[39] Rose writes, "But it is not the destiny of the biological citizen to be an isolated atom, at least in circumstances where the forms of life, ethical assumptions, types of politics, and communication technologies make new forms of collectivism possible."[40] Health advocacy and/or support organizations have the potential to become activist communities; formed around a shared disease, such communities are "frequently self-defined activist communities mobilized by the hope of a cure."[41] However, although many of these advocacy and/or support organizations define themselves as activist, the example of BCA provides a specific type of activism that may be particularly important to a new feminist health politics: an activist orientation that exists both alongside and in opposition to biomedicine. Simply put, BCA's activist orientation includes both a recognition of the promises of biomedicine and a recognition of its dangers. To maintain this dual stance, BCA explicitly rejects all funding from businesses and individuals that profit from the cancer industrial complex, including pharmaceutical corporations. Refusing funding from certain sources is clearly not feasible for every health advocacy or support organization, but two aspects of an activist orientation could be useful to groups even as they accept corporate sponsorship: a critical stance toward biomedical knowledge and a broad view of what constitutes women's health.

With the awareness of growing corporate influence in biomedicine, particularly the influence of "Big Pharma," one essential element of a new feminist health politics is a critical, perhaps watchdog, approach to biomedical knowledge. This approach acknowledges the significance of information created by biomedical experts (as opposed to, for example, the women's health movement's primary emphasis on experiential knowledge) but nevertheless positions activists as lay experts who, as biological citizens, are empowered to critique biomedicine. BCA's web site offers a list of "recent victories" that detail the group's no-holds-barred approach to challenging biomedical knowledge. In 2010, BCA successfully argued at an FDA hearing "to deny Genentech accelerated approval for TDM-1 for metastatic breast cancer patients based on one single-armed trial that has not given sufficient information on efficacy and safety."[42] Taking the stance that the drug approval process should not be so hasty as to approve drugs with no legitimate clinical benefit, BCA activists perform as well-informed, scientifically savvy advocates for women's health. Also in 2010, BCA formed its Screening Task Force to speak directly to the U.S. Preventive Services Task Force's new (2009) breast cancer screening guidelines.[43] BCA released its own screening recommendations that emphasized both the potential advantages and potential disadvantages of women under fifty having regular mammograms. BCA explains, "Women who are younger than age fifty and particularly concerned about breast cancer may wish to consider earlier mammography but should be aware of the higher risks of false positives, the reality that mammography is less effective in premenopausal women, and the risks of radiation from both screening and unnecessary treatment."[44] Rather than treating mammograms as a perfect tool for breast cancer detection, BCA embraces a more critical approach and suggests that women recognize the "pros and cons" of all breast cancer screening tools (including breast self-exams, clinical exams, and MRIs).

Although some of BCA's activism around issues of biomedical knowledge may seem reactive—that is, it reacted to Genentech's desire to receive early approval for its latest drug—I would suggest that BCA's critical/watchdog approach is actually active. BCA positions biological citizens as actively engaging with the knowledge produced by the biomedical industry. For BCA members, this means surveying recent news articles, reading scientific journals, and keeping track of drugs that are making their way through the FDA approval process. As active knowledge consumers and producers, BCA's leaders and members ultimately engage biomedicine in what I call "knowledge skirmishes" in which BCA challenges the value of biomedical tools for women. Olesen and Clarke suggest that "no knowledges are innocent, irrespective of the producers and their context, locus, or standpoint."[45] BCA produces knowledge—and challenges knowledge—based on a specific standpoint that privileges women's well-being over corporate profits. Furthermore, BCA's work aligns with the idea that more biomedicine is not always a good thing; that is, BCA takes part in what Clarke and colleagues describe as a "growing discourse attempting to articulate 'appropriate' levels and forms of biomedical intervention."[46] For example, in 2005 BCA began an online survey to collect information from women about their experiences with side effects while taking aromatase inhibitors (AIs). The results were published in 2008, with BCA noting "Here at BCA, we understand that patients often recognize emerging side effects before the medical community does. Through these reports, we hope to encourage additional research on the long-term side effects of AIs."[47] Although one might interpret much of BCA's work as directly opposing the biomedical industry, in this example BCA is both critiquing a treatment (aromatase inhibitors) and urging the biomedical establishment to do more research on the treatment. BCA's dual stance toward biomedicine is perhaps best summarized by its goals vis-à-vis the FDA: "Advocate for more effective and less toxic breast cancer treatments by shifting the balance of power in the Food and Drug Administration's drug approval process away from the pharmaceutical industry and toward the public interest."[48] While BCA is critical of the FDA's current procedures, it recognizes the need for better and more effective drugs that are approved through a standardized process (one that, in their vision, emphasizes the needs of people, not the needs of corporations).

BCA's ability to take a dual (and often critical) stance toward biomedicine is enhanced by its rejection of corporate sponsorship, and this rejection plays a substantial role in the second aspect of their activist orientation I wish to emphasize: its broad view of breast cancer. One of BCA's most well-known activist efforts is its "Think Before You Pink" campaign, which "calls for more transparency and accountability by companies that take part in breast cancer fundraising, and encourages consumers to ask critical questions about pink ribbon promotions."[49] The "Think Before You Pink" campaign speaks directly to the emphasis on women as consumers in postfeminist depictions of women's health. Whether women are deciding which drugs to take, which therapies to engage in, or which brand of yogurt to buy, postfeminist discourse often offers them empowerment through consumption. BCA's campaign addresses the consumer identity, but with a twist. BCA asks, if one is empowered through consumption, how can that empowerment be used not to meet individual needs (i.e., to treat an individual problem with an individual solution) but to meet collective needs (safety and efficacy in medical products, "truth" in advertising)? To this end, "Think Before You Pink" performs a rhetorical maneuver not unlike that of the consumer's rights movement, arguing for consumers' rights to knowledge about the products that they purchase.[50] However, while "Think" has certainly released information about "faulty goods" (in 2008, BCA focused its "Think" campaign on Yoplait's use of rBGH, or recombinant bovine growth hormone, in its yogurt products) and has successfully pressured corporations to change their products and/or advertising (Yoplait capitulated and removed rBGH), the "Think" campaign takes an additional—and pivotal—step: it asks consumers to engage in a broader understanding of the breast cancer industry, including the causes of breast cancer and potential preventive solutions.[51]

Over the years, "Think" has released a list of products that engage in pinkwashing, or the use of pink ribbons and breast cancer awareness themes to sell products that (may) contribute to causing breast cancer. In 2007, for example, "Think" focused on car manufacturers, identifying the toxic substances released in vehicle exhaust fumes and identifying the manufacturers (Ford, Mercedes, and BMW) that had pink campaigns.[52] Through its activism, BCA asks women to consider many difficult issues: What research, for example, will do the most good? How do we define good? What kind of awareness about breast cancer do we need when we are already aware that breast cancer is a problem? Ultimately, BCA's "Think" campaign asks individuals to act on a new perspective of women's health, a broad view of breast cancer. What I mean by this is multiple things, but perhaps most important is the sense that the broad view of breast cancer encompasses far more than a single woman's diagnosis and treatment decisions. The broad view places the woman in context and, in this case, asks her (and us) to see how everyday activities of purchasing yogurt, driving cars, or wearing makeup are part of the cancer industry. Understanding breast cancer with a broad view is what makes consumer choices relevant. Barbara Brenner, BCA's director, describes her broad view as a process of making connections during a TLC cancer tour in San Francisco: "I'm here because it's time, it's way past time for people concerned about cancer to start making connections. Connections between increasing incidents of many kinds of cancer—including my own kind of cancer, breast cancer—and equally scary, childhood cancers and what we as a society do to our air, our water, and our food supplies."[53] Importantly, BCA's broad view also encompasses issues that move beyond choices about consumption and focus specifically on issues of social inequality. BCA declares that it will "create awareness that it is not just genes, but social injustices—political, economic, and racial inequities— that lead to disparities in breast cancer outcomes."[54] The connections Brenner speaks of above are not merely between breast cancer and the environment but also between breast cancer and the experience of living in communities shaped by racism, sexism, classism, and homophobia.

The potential for all types of health advocacy and/or support organizations to be locations for an activist orientation that does not privilege the
interests of biomedicine but does not reject biomedicine either offers one
way for individuals as biological citizens to interact with biomedicine while
maintaining a critical stance in relation to the institutions and organizations
that shape new biotechnologies. Such an activist orientation may be easiest
for grassroots groups such as BCA that reject funding from the biomedical
industry at large, but it is certainly feasible that other groups could engage in
knowledge skirmishes and/or take a broad view of women's health. FORCE is
an excellent example of a biosocial community that focuses on women with
a genetic risk for breast cancer that also often functions to advocate for more
research funding and to help women living with the BRCA gene mutations.
However, there is a critical dimension to their work regarding some of the
knowledge produced by the biomedical industry. Their web site explains the
origins of the word "previvor" as a description for a woman who has a genetic
predisposition to cancer but has not been diagnosed with cancer: "The medical community uses the term 'unaffected carrier' to describe those who have
not had cancer but have a BRCA or other cancer-predisposing mutation. The
term applies from a medical perspective, but doesn't capture the experience
of those who face an increased risk for cancer and the need to make medical
management decisions."[55] In this case, the medical community is implicitly
critiqued for labeling women in a way that does not adequately capture the
breadth of their experiences.

I am not advocating that all health advocacy and/or support organizations
perform like BCA, but I am hoping that as one part of a new feminist health politics, we will recognize that many diverse organizations can play a pivotal role
in offering a critical stance toward the biomedical industry, one that does not
reject biomedicine but also does not unquestioningly embrace it. Ultimately,
emphasizing the activist potential of all types of health organizations offers
feminist activists one way to both disrupt some of the individualist rhetoric of
postfeminist women's health discourse (by emphasizing the biological collective) and construct and emphasize a critical dimension to women's consumption of medical services. Where many of the narratives in public discourse give
women little room to question biomedicine even as they are encouraged to
consume pharmaceuticals and other services, health advocacy and/or support
organizations that took a more critical stance would offer a vision of women as
critical consumers.

Health Inequalities

The broad view of breast cancer (and of women's health more generally) I described through BCA's "Think" campaign and its priorities (ensuring, for example, that medical research pays attention to social injustices) is an example of the second area of focus for a new feminist health politics: health inequalities. In the three case studies in this book, I pointed to the problems associated with representations of health that focus only on privileged individuals. Not only do such representations elide the very real health disparities that exist (for example, in the United States Hispanic women have the highest rate of cervical cancer, more than twice that of non-Hispanic white women), but they also paint a problematic picture of the face of any given disease (for example, white, heterosexual, middle-class women are given access to the language of postpartum disorders in a way that women of color, poor women, and lesbians are not).[56] By focusing on health inequalities, I hope to capture in this section the need for a feminist discourse on health disparities that moves beyond mere statistics. For example, why do Hispanic women have two times the incidence of cervical cancer? Why is cervical cancer stratified in the United States by race and class? The answers to these questions must move us beyond concerns about access to treatment, although such issues are important. Instead, discussions of health inequalities should cover a range of social and structural issues that relate to the development of disparities in health status among populations, including cultural differences, dimensions of social power, and hierarchies of race, class, and sex within the United States.

The concept of health disparities often refers to a broad area of concerns about differences in the incidence and prevalence of certain diseases and differences in mortality rates associated with particular diseases.[57] Health disparities in the United States are a historical phenomenon, and one avenue of understanding at least part of the cause of health disparities is to look to the history (and current workings) of the U.S. health care system. The U.S. health insurance market "developed as a primarily private, employment-based system" in the 1920s, despite the fact that European countries at the time were trending toward some form of nationalized health insurance.[58] Jonathan Cohn explains that in other industrialized countries in the 1920s and 1930s, health care was "on the way to becoming a right, rather than a privilege," while in the United States the privatization of health insurance created a hierarchy of access to health care: individuals with good insurance had access to care almost all the time, those with poor insurance had access only rarely or had but a portion of the care they needed, and those with no insurance either had no health care or had to rely on what charities were willing to provide.[59] The creation of the Medicare and Medicaid programs in 1965 alleviated some of the problems of the uninsured and underinsured, but the norm of private, employment-based health insurance went largely unchallenged. For many Americans, this system worked well (or well enough) through the early 1980s; the share of Americans with health insurance moved constantly upward from the 1940s through the 1970s, and by 1980, 90 percent of citizens were covered by health insurance.[60]

Contemporary conversations about health disparities often take place in the context of the biomedicalization era in which biomedical technology has proliferated but has also become far more expensive. By the mid-1980s, critics of the health industry were aware that the growing cost of health care was the beginning of a crisis. Cohn explains, "During the 1980s, large manufacturing companies, once the linchpin of the U.S. economy, were suddenly desperate to cut costs because they were struggling to keep up with foreign competitors who could produce goods more cheaply."[61] Their way to cut costs was to cut employee benefits, including health insurance. The most profitable companies in the 1990s were those that reduced costs by squeezing benefits (Walmart, for example, offered "skimpy benefits," and only to full-time workers who had been with the company for two years).[62] The number of Americans with health insurance declined precipitously, and the 1990s and 2000s were characterized by examples of individual financial devastation. By the 1990s medical debt was the leading cause of bankruptcy; a significant portion of bankruptcies were the result of "Americans without health insurance who ran up five-figure or six-figure hospital bills, sometimes during just one emergency or episode requiring intensive hospital care."[63] By 2008 there were forty-eight million uninsured Americans.[64] The increasing number of medical bankruptcies and the decreasing number of individuals with health insurance is but one aspect of the health care crisis that Americans faced in the first decade of the twenty-first century.

In the most recent wave of health care reform efforts (cumulating with the passage in 2010 of President Obama's Affordable Care Act), much attention was paid to the amount of money the United States was spending on health care. By 2010, national health spending was nearing 20 percent of U.S. GDP.[65] Sociologists Jacob Hacker and Theda Skocpol argue that deficit reduction has been a primary concern of politicians since the 1980s, and deficit reduction became a central feature in the debates about the Obama reforms. Deployed as a larger antigovernment strategy by conservatives, the deficit reduction frame called for cutting publicly funded health care to achieve a "less costly" and "less intrusive" government.[66] Although new reports suggested that the United

States was simply spending too much money on health care, an even larger problem loomed: despite the outflow of money for health care, the health of Americans consistently ranks poorly on a number of measures.[67] Physician Barbara Starfield describes the dynamic: "The high cost of the health care system is considered to be a deficit, but seems to be tolerated under the assumption that better health results from more expensive care."[68] However, the "better care" part of the equation is a myth; by 2000, in a ranking of thirteen industrialized countries on sixteen measures, the average rank of the United States was twelfth (including thirteenth for neonatal mortality and infant mortality and tenth for age-adjusted mortality).[69]

Starfield suggests that the explanation for poor health in the United States is "undoubtedly complex and multifactorial," but she points to three specific issues that should be addressed to positively change the health of all Americans: 1) the health care system; 2) the relationship between unintentional harmful effects (including adverse events caused by errors) and the type of care received; and 3) the relationships among income inequality, social disadvantage, and characteristics of health systems, including the relative contributions of primary care and specialty care.[70] The passage of Obama's health reforms in 2010 offers a partial answer to at least one of Starfield's issues: the Affordable Care Act should increase the number of insured individuals by requiring Americans to have health insurance coverage. This should add sixteen million people to Medicaid rolls, and the new law will subsidize private coverage for low- and middle-income people.[71] In addition, the government will monitor and regulate insurers more closely and will ban practices such as denial of care for preexisting conditions. I claim that this is a "partial" answer because the act does not achieve universal coverage (Americans reacted strongly against the idea of "socialized medicine") and, as physicians David Himmelstein and Steffie Woolhandler argue, the reform "will pump additional funds into the currently dysfunctional, market driven system, pushing up health costs that are already twice those in most other wealthy nations."[72] The recent Affordable Care Act attempts to answer the problem of access by supplying health insurance to more individuals; the assumption of the legislation is that unequal access to health care is one of the underlying causes of higher levels of disease and disability in certain populations.[73]

One of the risks of focusing health care reform solely on the issue of access to health care is similar to a key danger that haunts the inclusion-and-difference paradigm I discussed in the first chapter. That paradigm, which has driven much of the medical research since the late 1980s on differences in health status among population groups, can be understood as an attempt to answer the continuing problem of health disparities. Instead of looking at access as the central problem, the inclusion-and-difference paradigm looks at issues of appropriate inclusion within the medical arena. For example, new policies were created in the early 1990s to guarantee that more women and minorities would be included in clinical trials and as the targets of pharmaceutical drug development.[74] However, the inclusion-and-difference paradigm offers "inadequate intellectual resources" to challenge the perception that differences in health status (mortality rates, incidence rates) are not natural; that is, that differences are not simply a fact of biological difference.[75] Epstein explains, "Reformers who promoted inclusion pointed to health disparities—especially disparities by race—as part of the justification for changing biomedical research practices, but they did so typically without extended analysis of the complex array of conditions that might generate those disparities."[76] Likewise, while the recent efforts to reform health care seemed to focus on one structural issue—access—they did not engage in discussions of the complexity of issues behind health inequalities. Instead, most reform efforts have failed to bring adequate attention to the crucial set of issues behind health disparities, including "the ways in which inequalities and power differentials in the broader society affects people's exposure to health risks, their capacity to access quality medical care, and the likelihood that they will be subject to conscious or unconscious discriminatory treatment by health care professionals."[77]

I suggest that feminist health activists bring to the table intersectional models instead of biomedical, psychosocial, and biobehavorial models of health differences. In an extensive review of the differences between intersectionality and more standard approaches to the study of health disparities, Lynn Weber and Deborah Parra-Medina suggest that intersectional models have "great potential to provide new knowledge that can more effectively guide actions toward eliminating health disparities," in part because such models would draw from feminist work on intersectionality, which explicates the socially constructed and intricately intertwined nature of race, class, gender, and sexuality systems of social inequality."[78] In current feminist health activism, reproductive health is one area where an intersectional approach is making inroads in changing the nature of the discussions of health difference. By reproductive health, I mean far more than abortion rights. The list of commonly cited reproductive health disparities is lengthy and includes differences in cervical cancer rates (such as those I discussed above), infant mortality rates (African American, American Indian, and Puerto Rican infants have higher rates of mortality compared to white infants), maternal mortality rates (again, African American, American Indian, and Alaskan Native populations have higher rates), HIV/AIDS incidence rates (HIV is the third leading cause of death for African American women between twenty-five and forty-four), and STI incidence rates (as just one example, gonorrhea rates among African Americans are more than thirty times higher than that of whites and more than eleven times higher than that of Hispanics).[79] Feminist activists who draw upon an intersectional paradigm challenge two key aspects of reproductive health as popularly construed in the media: they challenge the language of choice that dominates some feminist discussions of reproductive health, and they move to expand our understanding of reproductive health beyond abortion.

Critiques of the choice paradigm with regard to abortion as it operated in the late twentieth century and early twenty-first century point in part to what Celeste Condit Railsback recognized about the original use of the term "choice" in the late 1970s: choice was intimately linked to individual freedom and thus became a limiting factor in the arguments abortion supporters could make.[80] Regarding public funding for abortion, for example, "Disputants who opposed public funding of abortions used the Pro-choice group's own ideograph, 'choice,' as an argument against requiring those who believed abortion to be immoral to pay for abortions through their taxes."[81] The severe limiting of public funds for abortion—including the passage of the Hyde Amendment—can be directly linked to the framing of abortion as an individual choice instead of a right.[82] Offering a more thorough critique of the neoliberal paradigm of choice, Andrea Smith argues that choice advocates often "take positions that are oppressive to women from marginalized communities."[83] For example, choice advocates have difficulty, according to Smith, taking a critical stance toward potentially dangerous contraceptives because the subject is reduced to whether or not women can choose to use them. Although serious safety issues are associated with Norplant and Depo-Provera and these contraceptives are marketed largely to minority populations, none of the mainstream pro-choice organizations have taken an explicit position on the need for informed consent.[84] Ultimately, arguments for choice regarding abortion ignore differences in women's ability to make a choice that are shaped by differences in access to safe abortion clinics and safe contraception. Furthermore, the language of choice ignores the underlying reasons for these differences in access, and the micro and macro structures of racism, sexism, and classism go unquestioned. The choice frame is patently elitist; the lives of white, upper-middle-class women are well represented, and the problems of all "others" disappear.

One example of intersectional activism that has already received some scholarly attention is the March for Women's Lives in Washington, D.C., in 2004. Communication scholar Sara Hayden argues that the march brought renewed vitality to the ideograph of choice because white women partnered with groups of women of color to focus on "broad-based demands for reproductive rights."[85] This partnering did not occur with ease; groups organized by women of color were not included in the in the early stages of planning for the march, originally titled the March for Freedom of Choice.[86] Faced with harsh criticism from a diverse group of organizations, the original sponsors of the march reorganized and a new title—the March for Women's Lives—was agreed upon. As Hayden notes, within the march the issue of choice did not disappear but became one of seven issues: choice, justice, access, health, abortion, global, and family planning.[87] The voices of women of color were particularly important in the re-creation, or revisioning, of choice: "Caricia Catalani of the National Latina Institute for Reproductive Health told the audience that she and other members of her community 'are here to remind everyone that choice means more than legal freedom. It means access to doctors. It means access to education. It means access to care in your language. We will have a choice when our communities survive.'"[88] Hayden suggests that as an "image event"—or an act of social protest intended to shape public opinion and designed for media dissemination—the March for Women's Lives (which had well over one million participants) had the power to revitalize choice by unmooring the ideograph of "choice" from its previous meanings and attaching it to a broader agenda.[89]

Although I partially agree with Hayden's assessment, I want to argue additionally that the more important rhetorical move of the march was the shifting of choice to one of many frameworks for understanding reproductive health. Several other frameworks—including the focus on saving women's lives and on justice—indicate the presence of an intersectional understanding of reproductive health. What is both enlightening and heartbreaking about the story of the march is the role of women of color, both their initial exclusion and their final inclusion. The sponsors of the march—the National Organization for Women, NARAL Pro-Choice, Planned Parenthood, and the Feminist Majority Foundation—were poised to replicate the postfeminist problem of focusing on white women with class privilege. Indeed, they would have replicated the problem, along with the insidious replication of a focus on neoliberal choice, had it not been for women's health activists of color. An intersectional perspective, then, requires women's health activists to engage in an explicit and ongoing integration of the lives and experiences of women who live outside of the idealized versions of womanhood that dominate postfeminist women's health discourse. That the largely white (dominant) feminist organizations had to be reminded of the importance of the diverse issues associated with women's health—the lives of women of color, lesbians, immigrant women, and so forth—is disheartening. In part, this problem suggests the continuation of a historical tension between women of color and the largely white feminist women's health establishment. These tensions exist despite extensive work in the 1980s and 1990s to integrate diverse perspectives into the movement, including the NWHN's two-year project on Black women's health that started in 1982 and the development of the National Black Women's Health Project (NBWHP) in 1984.[90] NBWHP member Sharon Gary-Smith explains that in the late 1980s, the "politics of health" for women of color always included the recognition that Black women faced "a multiplicity of issues—whether from racism and sexism, classism, or substandard housing, chronic financial limitations and unemployment."[91] Although she does not explicitly use the word "intersectional," Gary-Smith is pointing to an intersectional understanding of women's health that perceives women as existing within an interlocking matrix of domination in which race, class, gender and sexuality represent axes.[92]

This intersectional understanding of women's health is apparent in the communications of Loretta Ross (former director of NBWHP) to the Black women's health community. In an e-mail to the participants in the 2003 SisterSong conference (SisterSong defines itself as a "Women of Color reproductive justice collective"), Ross decried the lack of involvement of women of color in the march and reported that she had been belatedly invited to co-organize the march to ensure participation by women of color at every level. Ross focuses on the framework of the march—Freedom of Choice—as the primary problem. She explains that the pro-choice framework is too narrow because it speaks only to women with the ability to actually exercise reproductive choices. Ross argues, "This language [of choice] omits women who are poor, who are immigrants and refugees, women who are incarcerated or in the military, and women whose health services are provided or paid for by the government. In sum, it omits women who have few meaningful choices in their lives because of racism, xenophobia, homophobia, and poverty."[93] Ross and the SisterSong collective were remarkably successful in challenging the concept of choice and changing the face of the march. In a statement released in October 2003, the SisterSong collective made demands of the march organizers, which were largely met:

- Purposeful inclusion, from this day forward, of the complex diversity of women of color at various levels of decision making for the March.
- The intentional strategy to include a Women of Color schema that speaks to the lives of Women of Color and approved by Women of Color
- Interrogation of narrow, excluding language of Choice-only rhetoric that does not speak to the socio-historical and present day realities of Women of Color. We prefer the more inclusive language of human rights and reproductive rights.
- Demands that acknowledge a broader understanding of access issues (money, location, etc.) that discriminate against most women but disproportionately victimize Women of Color.[94]

The final demand in the list SisterSong created—that women's health activists "acknowledge a broader understanding of access issues"—is particularly interesting given my argument that an intersectional approach to health inequalities could be an important part a new feminist health politics. Although limited here to issues of access, SisterSong expanded their approach in later publications (their website and newsletters) into a call for justice.

At their National Conference in 2003, the members of SisterSong positioned themselves as outside the "mainstream abortion rights movement."[95] Over the course of several months, members of SisterSong (including Ross) held conference calls, convened plenary sessions at the conference, and mounted an e-mail campaign to discuss, question, and consider the role of women of color in the march. In its newsletters and web pages, SisterSong articulates a clear rhetoric of justice, a challenge to the rhetoric of choice that dominates not only postfeminist women's health discourse but also much of the current feminist discourse on reproduction. In one issue of the SisterSong newsletter, Asian Communities for Reproductive Justice offer this definition of reproductive justice: "Our vision of Reproductive Justice is the complete physical, mental, spiritual, political, economic, and social well-being of women and girls. Reproductive Justice states women's reproductive rights are human rights."[96] They continue, "We believe that Reproductive Justice will be achieved when women and girls have the economic, social and political power and resources to make healthy decisions about our bodies, sexuality and reproduction for ourselves, our families and our communities in all areas of our lives. For this to become reality, we need to make change on the individual, family, community and public and private institutional levels to end all forms of oppression."[97] The discourse of SisterSong positions justice as an understanding of women's health issues that necessarily takes into account the intersectional nature of oppression and domination.

The vision of justice SisterSong offers is just one approach to emphasizing the intersectional nature of women's health. In a feminist politics that concentrates on health inequalities rather than on health disparities, a topic that is often discussed outside of any context, such an approach is necessary. Weber and Parra-Medina suggest that an intersectional approach to understanding differences in health status differs in several important ways from biomedical, psychosocial, and biobehavioral paradigms. Three issues are particularly relevant to creating a feminist health politics that responds to public discourse about women's health that privileges a postfeminist erasure of health inequalities. First, where a biomedical paradigm fails to consider the social forces and contexts of women's lives, intersectional approaches "problematize the processes generating and maintaining the macro social structures of race, class, gender, and sexuality and seek to identify their relationships to individual and collective identities, behaviors, and health statuses.[98] Second, intersectional approaches privilege an understanding of power as relational rather than distributional (a relational approach examines relations of dominance and subordination among groups).[99] Third, instead of beginning with the experiences and statistics associated with dominant groups, an intersectional approach "emerges from the perspectives of multiply oppressed groups, especially women of color, so that women of color serve as the reference point, and their health is examined in its own context, not as it deviates from the white norm."[100] As part of a new feminist health politics, embracing an intersectional perspective begins with a recognition of health inequalities, includes a critique of such inequalities through an intersectional approach (focusing on social structures, understanding power as relational, and emerging from the perspectives of individuals outside the dominant group), and ends with solutions that focus not only on the individual but also on the larger culture. As Weber and Parra-Medina explain, "Many of the actions necessary to eliminate health disparities will require strategies that involve changing social structures in sectors other than health."[101] Focusing on health inequalities is one partial correction to the invisibility of "other" women—those who fall outside a white, heterosexual, middle-class norm—in postfeminist narratives about women's health. Further, such a focus also challenges mainstream biomedical disparities research that all too often decontextualizes statistical evidence about health differences among individuals and populations.

The Politics of Gender

As a third area of focus for a new feminist health politics I suggest that feminist activists should actively critique the often-outdated gendered assumptions that guide postfeminist health narratives. The public narratives I have analyzed in this book reduce complex stories of women, risk, and illness into a narrative that positions women as needing to take care of their health for the sake of others (their children or spouses) and not for their own sake. In other words, one feature of women's experiences that is made salient by postfeminist narratives of women's health is women's roles as mothers and wives. Indeed, representations of women that reified compulsory heterosexuality and a larger heterosexual matrix guided each of the public narratives about women's health in this book. The narratives I analyzed made heterosexual relationships and a singular understanding of "proper" womanhood natural; the contingencies of what it might mean to be a mother or to be a woman with cancer are absent. Instead, what appears is a very specific a view of "gender coherence whereby what a person feels, how a person acts, and how a person expresses herself sexually is the articulation and consummation of a gender."[102] Each of the narratives features women in relationships (or hoping to be in relationships) with men; their heterosexual relationships (including the nuclear family) are part of what makes them women. A new feminist health politics must pay attention to the issue of gender.

Feminist health activists can draw upon a range of theories about gender, gender construction, and gender roles. Because I see the three areas of focus I am presenting (activism and advocacy communities, health inequalities, and gender politics) as complex, dynamic areas of focus that encompass a range of stances and potential theoretical alignments, I do not wish to endorse only one theory of gender at this point. However, it is useful to recognize that the alignment of postfeminist and neoliberal discourses in the women's health arena has created a situation in which gender, and more specifically, traditional understandings of womanhood, is an explicit factor in the public constructions of meanings for health. This is an issue that scholars in several areas have pointed to, albeit obliquely. Steven Epstein, for example, writes extensively about the emergence of sex-based differences as one of the foundations upon which the inclusion-and-difference paradigm is built. Assuming the presence of sex-based difference (and, for that matter, race-based difference) "has presupposed a forgetting of feminist critiques of much previous research into sex differences," including the problems of essentialism posed by sex-based biology.[103] Epstein explains one part of the sex difference conundrum: "Sex categories have an obvious biological grounding in the body. But the precise ways in which sexed bodies correspond to our social categories—or fail to do so—are obscured by an overwhelmingly strong ideology of sexual dimorphism: the belief that males and females are utterly distinct, if not opposite, and that no middle ground exists."[104] Epstein's reflections are largely focused on how an ideology of sexual dimorphism plays out in medical research, but my point is slightly different. In mainstream public discourse—not medical discourse—about women's health, sex based differences play out on the field of gender differences. It is not just that public discourse assumes biological differences but also that those biological differences are innately related to differences in gender: a female is a woman, a male is a man, and there are certain ways of being a woman and a man that are identified (and reified) as normal.

Scholarly work that focuses explicitly on constructions of gender and risk come closer to my point about public discourse. Kelly Hannah-Moffat and Pat O'Malley suggest that gender and risk are mutually constituted: "Gendered knowledges, norms and hierarchies are linked with understandings of what constitutes a risk; the tolerance level of risk; the extent to which risk consciousness will be accepted or denied in public discourse or self-image; and whether risks are to be avoided and feared, regarded as just one of the costs of a certain lifestyle, or even valued as an experience and valorized as an opportunity for displays of courage and strength."[105] As just one example, Hannah-Moffat and O'Malley point to the discourses about pregnancy in which "risk techniques have played a key role in shifting attention to the foetus and to the responsibility of the mother in becoming knowledgeable and competent regarding risks to her baby."[106] The emphasis on a mother's responsibility overlaps with, and indeed in some cases has the potential to expand, ideologies of motherhood in which women's selfless care-giving attributes are naturalized (in this case through holding women fully responsible for the production of a healthy infant and the raising of a healthy child). If, within the domain of risk, "gender can be constituted, reconstituted, or erased," then considerations of how gender is constituted in public discourse about women's health are important.[107] I have argued that in relation to the risks breast cancer, postpartum depression, and cervical cancer pose, gender—namely, femininity—is constructed largely through a reification of discourses of traditional womanhood. This trend of returning to elements of traditional womanhood may be most clear in mainstream public discourse, although I suspect that research on medical discourse would point to a similar trend.

One area where feminist health activists are actively responding to the reification of traditional gender norms is sex education. Contemporary sex education aligns with the politically conservative abstinence-only movement; sex education programs stress moral character and values but ignore contraception and safer sex techniques and condemn sexual behavior outside heterosexual marriage. The web site Scarleteen: Sex Education for the Real World promotes sexual self-determination for teens and refutes, refuses, and reframes traditional gender roles. Scarleteen declares the need for its web site by citing statistics (for pregnancy, STIs, and so forth), but also by positioning the web site as an important resource for teenagers who may be receiving little sex education in schools or homes because of what it carefully describes as "cultural contexts and politics" that have reduced "teen and young adult access to sound, accurate, comprehensive and inclusive sex education."[108] Scarleteen is not new—it was founded in 1998—but it provides a plethora of up-to-date resources on sexuality, sexually transmitted infections, and basic information about things such as genitalia and menstrual cycles. What unites the information offered on Scarleteen is what founder Heather Corinna describes as a feminist perspective on sex education, a perspective that emphasizes two themes: self-determination and gender as a construction, not a biological fact. Several of her points are worth quoting in full. Feminist sex education

- Emphasizes—for all sexes and genders, not just one or two—autonomy, personal responsibility, full and active consent, sexuality in the holistic context of a whole, well-rounded life and healthy, equitable relationships, self-esteem, nonsubordination and nonviolence, safety, health, happiness and pleasure and very real equality in sexuality, in which equal voice and accord are given to and issues from any and all partners in sexual partnerships and sexual activity.
- Does not treat gender or sex as binary, and acknowledges gender as constructed, not essential, biological or assigned and sex as an often-problematic distinction.
- Recognizes the strong and pervasive effect of cultural and personal sex and gender roles on the individual and interpersonal sexuality, and educates readers about those roles and their right to choose sex and gender roles which are desired, not merely assigned. Addresses cultural inequalities of sex and gender which effect sexuality, such as the effects of commodifying women's bodies, the glorification of sexual violence, objectification, other minorities and sexuality in the media,

economic divides, the greater sexual burdens some groups bear, the greater rates of sexual abuse and rape among some groups, as well as the detrimental effects of patriarchy upon men, male sexuality, identity and relationships.[109]

Corinna's description about gender as a construction ultimately places gender (and sexual decision making) within the larger context of patriarchal power relations. Although she does not say so explicitly, part of what Corinna is pointing to is akin to my discussion of the intersectional perspective of health inequalities in which power is understood to be relational. Such an approach recognizes that "race, class, gender, and sexuality are systems of power relationships among groups, where one group or groups hold power over others and uses that power to secure material resources—such as wealth, income, or access to health care and to education."[110] In the case of sex education, traditional gender roles have been frequently used in public discourse as a way to refuse teenagers, especially young women, access to sexual knowledge.

Corinna's—and the web site's—focus on sexual self-determination (at points, Corinna suggests that individuals have an inalienable right to their own body) is always linked to a steadfast refusal and critique of traditional gender roles. In an extensive interview, Hanne Blank, author of *Virgin: The Untouched History*, and Scarleteen carefully depict virginity through a political lens. Blank argues that virginity has long been depicted as a central life issue for women, not men. She explains, "For much of human history, a woman's life was literally at the mercy of virginity. A woman who lost her virginity before she married was pretty much doomed: she was dishonored, her family was disgraced by her, it was likely that no one would be willing to marry her, and she might be beaten or even killed by her family. This was true whether she had lost her virginity voluntarily or been raped—it didn't matter."[111] This perspective on virginity points to the construction of the sexually pure good woman, and Blank follows it with a full-fledged critique. Although she notes that the concept of virginity itself might not be harmful in and of itself (that is, if virginity is simply used as a descriptive—not a moral—term to designate a sexual status), in lived contexts, the concept of virginity has been quite harmful: "If what you mean by 'virginity' is 'a particular quality that women have to have or else we kill them,' I'd say that's pretty harmful. Or if what you mean by 'virginity' is 'people who haven't had sex are better and nicer and shinier than people who have had sex,' I think that's harmful, too, because sexual history is a pretty flimsy basis on which to decide that some people are better human beings than others."[112]

As a web site that offers information about sex and sexuality to teens, Corinna and the Scarleteen staff not only disrupt and refute traditional gender roles for women and men (the content includes substantial amounts of information about diverse sexual and gender roles), they also challenge the hysteria found in popular culture about teenagers and sex. Navigating carefully around the issue of age, the Scarleteen web site promises to offer "respectful messaging encouraging critical thought, self-care and care for others, rather than shame or fear, which suggests and supports non-participation in sexual activities until such a time or a situation in which an individual wants to participate in those activities for themselves; until an individual feels prepared to manage and handle them well, including care for physical and mental health, adequate assertiveness and esteem and the ability to recognize and enact the import of mutual consent and benefit."[113] Importantly, the decision to engage in sexual activity is made by the individual, not by society or by Scarleteen's staff. Certainly human sexuality "poses both potential benefits as well as potential detriments," and Scarleteen's stance is to work to provide information to help teens "sustain [their] sexual well-being."[114] In the end, youth sexuality (described as sexuality of people under eighteen—the current legal majority) "poses no real threat to us when it is entered into and developed responsibly and compassionately."[115]

As an example of feminist health activism that actively engages in the politics of gender that underlie much of public discourse about women's health, Scarleteen is promising but also open to critique on a number of fronts. Scarleteen's mode of critiquing traditional gender roles often relies on a liberal notion of self-determination and bodily ownership that treats the body as property and the individual as rational and autonomous. Both of these ideas are problematic, especially in a feminist health politics that could work to emphasize intersecting relationships (the relational aspects of health inequalities, the communities constructed through citizens sharing a health problem) and responds to public discourse in which the self and the body are not depicted as fixed but as dynamic and mutable. Further, without critically engaging the social and institutional structures that enable one to enact bodily self-determination, the ideal of bodily ownership (and the supposed freedom that comes with owning one's body) Scarleteen presents assumes that all young women and men have an equal opportunity to make decisions about their bodies.[116] However, I offer Scarleteen as an example of feminist activism in same mode as the examples of SisterSong and BCA; none of these examples are critique-proof, but all of them illuminate potential areas of focus for a new feminist health politics. Women's health in this historical moment is "beset by dilemmas, paradoxes, and contradictions—in both feminist theorizing and women's health situations—which cannot be ignored."[117] Instead of reducing or constraining women's health agendas and theoretical lenses, the best approach to a complex situation may be to encourage many agendas and many theoretical lenses. The three areas of potential focus for a new feminist health politics that I have outlined—the promise of activism in health advocacy and/or support organizations, health inequalities, and gender politics—are one way to reconceptualize women's health within the rapidly changing world of biomedicine and the neoliberal and postfeminist meanings created for women's health in mainstream public discourse.

Proliferating Narratives and Subjectivities

Near the end of an article about the ways women have voluntarily adopted practices of self-surveillance and self-governance in relation to breast cancer risk, Jessica Polzer and Ann Robertson draw an interesting conclusion: "It is reasonable to assert, then, that the women's health movement, which openly encouraged women to become more knowledgeable about their bodies, has provided a fertile ground for a neoliberal mode of genetic governance to take hold and have meaning in women's everyday lives. Within the politics of health of the twenty-first century, women are increasingly called upon to take charge of their health through acts of "choice" and self-regulation."[118] The fertile ground of knowledge to which Polzer and Robertson refer is now part of the complex landscape of women's health on which feminist interventions can actively engage. In this project, I have focused on one aspect of the broad landscape of knowledge—the meanings made for women and women's health in mainstream public discourse. Between the representations of women's lives in the media (often of celebrities' lives) and feminist activist approaches to women's health are a multitude of other spheres of meaning, including women's lived experiences and personal medical encounters and the biomedical discourse of medical research. Nevertheless, how women are positioned in public discourse is significant because identities such as the cancer/risk-free woman and the risky mother offer models for understanding a life situation that provide guidelines for how to feel, act, and live with a particular illness. Our understandings of ourselves and our lives are developed in concert with the narratives that populate public discourse.

Social movement scholar James Darsey offers a useful approach to the idea of progress in social movements: defined rhetorically, progress means "rendering unnecessary the expenditure of argumentative energy or attention on certain claims."[119] The women's health movement has had substantial success in rendering unnecessary time spent on arguing, for example, for the need for medical research about women's health or the need to include women in clinical studies. Indeed, arguments of this type have been so successful they have contributed to constructing the (at times problematic) inclusion-and-difference paradigm that now guides much of medical research. Ultimately, arguments for the need to pay attention to difference are now common sense, although professional advocacy groups will continue to advocate for particular trials and types of research. In addition to the need for new areas of focus in a new feminist health politics, contemporary feminist health politics can (and should) be responsive to public discourse in a very specific way. Namely, feminist health activists—whether in the context of a grassroots organization such as BCA or online in forums such as the Scarleteen web site—can participate in constructing alternative public narratives about women's health and thus alternative subjectivities for women.

Part of the problem with mainstream public narratives about women's health is that they offer a largely unified understanding of womanhood through the identity of the vulnerable empowered woman. While I have offered multiple critiques of this particular representation of womanhood, perhaps the most significant problem is the vulnerable empowered woman's hegemonic status. Alternative representations of women, the relationships of women to health and disease, and women's position in relation to the biomedical establishment, are difficult to find in mainstream public discourse, whether on the nightly news or in celebrity gossip magazines. The solution is not a closing of the public discourse about women's health but rather the creation by feminist health activists of a broader and more diverse range of stories. Clarke and Olesen argue that "the [modern] destabilization of individual identity and subjectivity allowed space and place for multiple selves (rather than one authentic version and a series of false faces) and multiply experienced selves, subjectivities based on multiple selves, multiple subject positionings in the heterogeneous cartographies of contemporary life."[120] A new feminist health politics can contribute to this explosion of subjectivities by expanding, not limiting, the narratives about women's health. In their lived experiences, women may interact with the narratives of women's health—and the subjectivities offered—in public discourse in a variety of ways, perhaps taking what is meaningful or what aligns with their experience and applying it to their own lives, perhaps resisting the relatively limiting subjectivity of the vulnerable empowered woman, or perhaps accepting that subjectivity as a model for behavior, emotions, and expectations.

Narratives can be tools for understanding and working through life situations; my goal for a new feminist health politics is to offer women as many tools, as many narratives, as possible.

As just one example of how a proliferation of narratives could offer women different subjectivities, different tools for living, consider the recasting of the issue of vulnerability in the examples of feminist activism I have offered above. Women's vulnerability in postfeminist discourse is largely painted through discussions of risk. Over the course of this book, I have offered glimpses of what risks women are depicted as encountering in narratives about women's health. Women are "at risk" from a variety of external and internal factors—lifestyle issues, genetic issues, and even (in the case of the at-risky/risky young woman) women's propensity toward risky sexual behavior. In part because postfeminist discourse reifies (and reinvigorates) gender stereotypes and traditional gender roles, a woman's vulnerability can be traced back to her own genetic flaws, her own mysterious hormonal systems, and her own behavioral and emotional irrationality. Thus, the largest risk faced by women is a risk they cannot avoid: the risk of being a woman.

A new feminist health politics focusing on health inequalities, gender politics, and the activist potential of health organizations can offer a significantly different construal of vulnerability and empowerment. Although statistics regarding individual risk are deployed in the examples of feminist activism I discussed above, they are often deployed under a larger umbrella of justice that moves perceptions of the source of women's vulnerability from internal to external. By external I mean social and political factors, not lifestyle factors. The Scarleteen web site, for example, gives many examples of statistics that indicate risk. In a section called "The STI Files," Scarleteen offers this observation regarding HPV: "As many as one in ten Americans have HPV, and some studies show that at least one-third of all sexually active young adult have genital HPV infections. It is often stated that more than half of all college-age women will become infected with HPV during their college career, and many sexual healthcare providers consider that HPV is simply a symptom of people being sexually active, because it's just that common."[121] The discussion of HPV acknowledges that the best way to prevent HPV is to avoid genital contact with partners, but it does not engage in any discussion of promiscuity and offers detailed information about the use of condoms as one way to reduce the risk of contracting HPV.

The "STI Files" offer similar information about herpes, HIV/AIDS, and nearly every other possible STI. This information certainly offers individual readers a chance to assess their risk of contracting an STI based on their own sexual behavior, but such risks do not exist alone in depictions of vulnerability. In an article titled "I Guess You Just Have to Be Prepared to Die!" (the link for this article is featured on the site's STI pages), founder Heather Corinna offers a critique of an abstinence-only film called *No Second Chance*.[122] The title of her article is the verbatim response offered by one of the characters in the film to the question, "What if I want to have sex before I get married?" Corinna's critique of the link between sex and death is thorough, and she offers an extensive reading of statistics from the Centers for Disease Control that point to exactly why sex in and of itself is not causing death. Her conclusion implicitly points to an entirely different area of vulnerability: misinformation.

> Now that we've got all that sorted: by all means, having sex can result in some health issues or conditions (and some of them certainly are or can become serious) and can be related directly to a death. . . . But. You are much less likely to die from sex than you are from a whole host of other behaviours or circumstances, some of which the same folks would not warn you about with anything close to the same urgency or intensity. I just don't see driver's ed teachers telling you that if you get in a car at all, you need to be "prepared to die," even though more people die in car accidents than those who die as a result of having any kind of sex. (I also don't imagine they say that not wearing a seatbelt when you are in a car is playing "Russian roulette.") . . . Anyone who is stating or making it sound like sex or premarital sex is something more likely to kill you than anything else is being baldly dishonest. Whether you have sex with a partner in or out of marriage, with a partner of any given gender, at any given age and even IF (though we don't advise it) you take risks with your health and don't have sex safely, it is not, by any stretch, highly likely to kill you, and you do NOT have to "be prepared to die" if you choose to be sexually active. Not any more than you need to be prepared to die because we're all going to freaking die at some point no matter what we do, anyway.[123]

Although Corinna recognizes that sex carries some risk, she positions the bald lies of the abstinence-only film as increasing the vulnerability of teenagers.

This type of external vulnerability is linked not only to misinformation but also to the political values of those who offer the information and the system that supports those values. As Corinna notes, such dishonesty is especially problematic because "they're telling you that they're trying to scare the crap out of you expressly out of concern for your health, rather than because they want you to conform to their own personal set of values."[124] Although this particular example focuses on information, the "Think" campaign as well as the revision of the March for Choice to the March for Women's Lives push this outward understanding of vulnerability even further, linking women's health to how they are systemically vulnerable. BCA's most recent "Think" campaign focuses on the pharmaceutical company Eli Lilly's production of rBGH. In BCA's "Stop Milking Cancer" campaign, Eli Lilly is depicted as the cause of women's vulnerability to cancer: "Eli Lilly has taken pinkwashing to a whole new level. By adding rBGH to the products they sell, Eli Lilly has completed its cancer profit circle: it creates cancer with rBGH, it sells cancer treatment drugs like Gemzar, and it sells a drug, Evista, to reduce the risk of breast cancer in women at high risk of the disease. Eli Lilly's cancer drugs made $2,683,000,000 for the company in 2008. Its potentially carcinogenic dairy hormone made $985,000,000 in the same year. Eli Lilly is milking cancer."[125] Positioned as the potential victims of Eli Lilly's cancer cycle, women are urged to recognize the problem with Lilly's use of rBGH and the larger problems of a for-profit medical and pharmaceutical industry.

Because the concept of systemic vulnerability focuses on systemic sources of vulnerability—prompted by a larger critique of classism, racism, sexism, homophobia, and (often) capitalism—it has a clear link to social justice movements. This link is directly acknowledged in BCA's second and third priorities, which call for people to use a social justice lens—focusing on political, economic, and racial inequalities—to understand breast cancer.[126] As framed through BCA's rhetoric, for individuals vulnerable to systemic problems, empowerment and change does not come from focusing on the self. Following a neoliberal path, the postfeminist vulnerable empowered woman experiences both vulnerability and empowerment as self-focused. A re-visioning of vulnerability as a systemic phenomenon likewise promotes an understanding of empowerment as necessarily outside the self. Through the social justice frame deployed by BCA, SisterSong and Scarleteen, empowerment includes linking personal, organizational, and social change. Ester Shapiro describes these linkages as "'virtuous circles' that expand women's empowerment."[127] Understanding empowerment as "circling" prompts attention to "the flow of power/empowerment [that] travels between individuals, groups and institutions, and thus toward linking gains at the macro-institutional level with real changes in the everyday lives of women in different social contexts."[128] BCA's web site offers one interpretation on the circling of empowerment: "We pledge to continue to encourage our members to both ask tough questions and to understand the connections between what they can do personally and the social changes that are needed to end the breast cancer epidemic."[129]

A feminist health politics that engages in the proliferation of narratives has the potential to change how we live our lives in part because it offers a revisioning of both vulnerability and empowerment. The examples of Scarleteen, BCA, and SisterSong can certainly be critiqued from a number of standpoints, but each works to position women differently—and offers women different ways to make sense of their lives—than the postfeminist narratives of women's health. These three organizations are not the only sources of alternative subjectivities. Throughout the case studies, I referred on occasion to feminist interpretations of the health issues at hand: the feminist activists and psychologists who insist on looking at constructs of motherhood when considering postpartum depression, the writers for *Bitch* magazine who voiced concern about the exclusionary potential of the depictions of the "Gardasil girl," and the feminist activists (such as those of BCA) who declare, in opposition to the optimistic narratives of mainstream breast cancer culture, that "cancer sucks." Each of these examples takes part in constructing a different narrative about women and health, often narratives in which women are connected to each other (across, through, and around differences of race, class, and sexuality), to their environment (their social, political, institutional environment as well as the earth itself), to their families and friends, to their bodies, and to the findings of biomedical science. However, the many different subjectivities for women that feminist activists have constructed currently exist on the edge of mainstream public discourse; these are narratives and identities that are part of the counterpublic that presses against and challenges mainstream postfeminist discourse. The challenge feminist health activists now face is exactly how to engage postfeminist, neoliberal constructions in mainstream discourse when feminists and feminist perspectives are routinely excluded from (or tokenized within) mainstream media.

Afterword

From Margin to Center

I care deeply about women's health. As I was writing the preceding chapters, I reflected on the many ways my life—my happiness, security, and well-being—rests upon the health and well-being of the women around me. Perhaps more than anyone else, my mother's experiences have guided my interests and my passion—her memories of an unexpected postpartum hemorrhage after my birth, the surprise of finding a lump in her breast a few short months after a clean mammogram, and the experience of breast cancer from surgery to chemotherapy to radiation and beyond—but other women are central as well. I have watched friends grapple with cancer, with pregnancy and childbirth, with sexually transmitted infections and broader issues of sexuality, and with body image and dieting. My approach to studying women's health is not focused on policy making or the minute details of medical research. Rather, I want to understand how we—myself, my friends, my family, and millions of Americans—understand and make sense of women's health issues. In my analysis of mainstream public discourse, I have argued that our current understandings are problematic on at least four levels—the focus on elite women, the reification of traditional gender roles, the depoliticization of women's health, and the unquestioning acceptance of biomedicine. I concluded by suggesting that feminist discourse can offer new compelling alternative subjectivities to the vulnerable empowered woman of postfeminist discourse by encouraging a proliferation of narratives about women's health. My hope is that the future holds a centering of women's health discourse on subjectivities that represent women challenging, not acquiescing to, the power of biomedicine and traditional gender roles. But how does one move feminist representations of women's health from the margin to the center? Below, I offer a series of thoughts, questions, and prompts that point to possible pragmatic strategies for transforming mainstream public discourse.

The media are important. The story of the 2004 March for Women's Lives is significant for numerous reasons. As I have already discussed, the march holds important lessons for women's health activists about the need to centralize the experiences of many women, not just white, middle-class women. Another lesson of the march relates directly to the media. Fair.org, a national media watchdog, reported soon after the march that the media had paid little attention to the march. The three national broadcast networks aired a combined total of eight stories about it, compared to their extensive coverage of a Promise Keepers march in 1997, which garnered twenty-six stories.[1] This was a significant moment in the fight for women's health care, and the coverage was sparse at best. Numerous factors may have played into the lack of coverage, including the possibility that reproductive justice was not a politically "hot" issue in 2004. Indeed, the reporters covering the march voiced this opinion; CNN's Elaine Quijano reported, "This election year, each group hopes to spark renewed interest, enough to have an impact at the ballot box. But political analysts say more than three decades after Roe v. Wade, most voters have already made up their minds."[2] For future rallies, marches, and other examples of mass protest focused on women's health, organizers would do well to make a concerted effort to ensure media coverage. What events might attract the attention of the media? What ideas or concepts make good sound bites? Social change depends upon the sharing of information, and without media attention, the knowledge crafted by the marchers in 2004 was shared with only a small segment of the American public.

Language matters. As a rhetorical scholar I often take this issue for granted, but it is worth stating that the words we use carry meanings for the world. Strategically thinking about language regarding women's health should be part of moving a feminist perspective on women's health to the center of public discourse. For example, I suggested in my analysis of postpartum depression narratives that constructions of motherhood play an important role in normalizing the distress (elite) women feel as mothers. Changing parenting practices to include more social support for mothers, better maternity leave, and so forth could start with changing how we describe both mothering and fathering in our everyday conversations. One example of how to change our language can be found on the MomsRising website, a "network of people just like you, united by the goal of building a more family-friendly America."[3] On its home page, MomsRising contains prominent links to eight areas of concern: health care, paid family leave, early learning/child care, toxics, afterschool/TV, paid sick days, fair pay, and flexible work. Many of these issues are particular to women in the work force. However, MomsRising frames the issues in gender-neutral terms (paid family leave, and elsewhere paid "maternity and paternity leave") that supports active parenting by individuals of all sexes.[4]

Men's health is a feminist issue. Men played an important role in each of the case studies of this book, often as spouses or fathers, but also occasionally as individuals facing the same health risks. The example of HPV and cervical cancer is particularly interesting because HPV is a virus that both men and women can receive, and it causes cancer in both sexes. Yet when Gardasil was originally approved by the FDA, it was approved for women only. Even when men were added to the FDA approval, the recommendations of the Centers for Disease Control were less forceful for men (they "permit" the vaccination for men but "recommend" it for women).[5] The unequal status of men and women in public discourse about HPV and in the policies regarding the vaccination signals a continuation of the focus of processes of medicalization and regulation on women's bodies. Sociologist Patricia Reiker explains the need for feminists to engage in men's health: "Feminists have a vested interest in advocating for policies and circumstances around the world that shape men's ability to develop healthy sex lives, which, by definition, has to include respect for the rights of those with whom they partner, regardless of gender."[6] Reiker's point can be expanded: feminists have a vested interest in men's health both in and out of the sexual arena. Men, like women, can have breast cancer, postpartum depression, and HPV. Granted, some diseases are sex specific (ovarian cancer, testicular cancer), but including men in the public conversation about diseases that cross the sex boundary may very well change the entire structure of the narrative.

Find allies in unexpected places. Although much of feminist activism on women's health has occurred outside the biomedical industry (women's health advocates have prized laypeople's opinions and critiques), finding allies within the medical industry is one way to move the feminist perspective on women's health from margin to center. The increasing number of women physicians has been a key to the success of women's health centers linked with academic health centers. Donna Shelley argues that "today, the women's health movement is strongly influenced by the increased number of women physicians," many of whom take a woman-centered approach to health care that emphasizes "mutual respect and shared decision making between physician and patient,

comprehensive care delivered by a multidisciplinary team of health professionals, continuing education of patients and physicians that incorporates gender-
and sex-specific knowledge, and a commitment to quality assurance."[7] However,
moving even further afield than the focus on women physicians, I suggest that
one arena of potential alliances could be the growing movement to redefine "professionalism" for all physicians. Stephen Cha and colleagues report that "in a
recent joint statement, the American Board of Internal Medicine, the American
College of Physicians, and the European Federation of Internal Medicine defined
professionalism using the principles of social justice, patient welfare, and patient
autonomy, calling on physicians to be 'activist in reforming health care systems.'"[8]
With this statement in mind, Dr. Cha and numerous other medical practitioners
have created "activism courses" designed for medical students. These courses
focus on creating change in both patients' lives and health policy.[9] Encouraging
specifically feminist health activism through medical activism courses would
bring the feminist perspective on women's health care (and, frankly, all health
care) to a new audience of medical students.

Think globally, act locally. Acting locally is certainly one of the standard
calls of social activism (even Scarleteen's Corinna encourages readers to "act
locally" for causes they feel passionate about). What might acting locally for
women's health from a feminist activist perspective look like? Shelly Blair is a
graduate student working on her Ph.D. in the Department of Communication
at Texas A&M University. Over the past few years, Blair has ensconced herself
in the "Aggieland" community. She volunteers at the Planned Parenthood in
Bryan, Texas, as a patient escort. She writes about local and national events on
her blog, Fair and Feminist. With another graduate student, Vandhana Ramadu-
rai, she produces and hosts a local radio show, also titled *Fair and Feminist*.
With the blog and radio show, Blair has created the space to talk about women's
health and a variety of other feminist issues, and she is active with those issues
through her volunteering. Acting locally for Blair is a significant contribution
in part because of the context in which she works. Bryan's Planned Parenthood
is nationally known for the pro-life demonstrations it has inspired, including
the now-national "40 Days for Life" campaign. In a dominantly conservative
community, the besieged Planned Parenthood stands behind wrought-iron
fences and gates. The presence of Blair and other patient escorts reaffirms the
vital (and yet, in this community, often invisible) presence of activists working
for women-centered health care.

Engage in national healthcare politics. I have offered in this afterword a few
thoughts regarding possible directions for change that could bring a feminist

perspective on women's health to the center of public discourse: revitalizing activists' connections to media (the meaning-makers of our contemporary society), focusing on the language we use to describe women's health issues, recognizing that men's and women's health issues are often intertwined, creating alliances with diverse groups (such as medical students), and emphasizing the necessity of acting locally in our own communities. One final issue deserves attention, and that is the necessity for feminists to continue to engage on a national and state level with the politics of health care.

Feminist organizations were active in the 2009–2010 health care reform debates. As just one example, in January 2010, a group of women's health and feminist organizations that included Raising Women's Voices (a feminist collaborative made up of the National Women's Health Organization, the Avery Institute for Social Change, and the MergerWatch Project); Our Bodies, Ourselves; and Women of Color United for Health Reform sent an open letter to House Speaker Nancy Pelosi and Senate Majority Leader Harry Reid with recommendations regarding women's health for the final reform bill.[10] In addition to arguing for the removal of the anti-abortion Stupak Amendment, the organizations also recommended "a requirement that women's preventive health services and screenings be covered without co-pays or deductibles; coverage of more people through expansion of Medicaid eligibility; establishment of an 'exchange'; coverage for legal immigrants without a five-year waiting period; and making coverage more affordable while keeping penalties for violating coverage mandates less burdensome for low-income people."[11] While the final version of the Affordable Care Act did not include all of these suggestions, some were clearly present and the Stupak anti-abortion amendment was not included in the bill.

One significant problem related to feminist action in national and state health politics is its invisibility. In the case of the letter to Pelosi and Reid, only progressive web sites offered coverage, and most of those sites were related in some way to the letter's writers (thus, the Our Bodies, Ourselves collective covered the letter in a blog posting on Our Bodies, Our Blog). More recently, in the spring of 2011, a feminist perspective on the plans to defund Planned Parenthood at the national level was slightly more visible: mainstream news organizations used sources such as NARAL Pro-Choice America president Nancy Keegan and reported that Republicans were enacting a "vendetta against Planned Parenthood."[12] Making sure that a feminist perspective on national health debates is visible leads us back to where I began this afterword—recognizing that media matters and developing productive relationships with national news forums.

Bringing a feminist perspective to bear on national and state-level health politics is significant just now because while the Affordable Care Act passed in 2010 and has yet to be repealed, health inequalities continue to be a pressing problem. At the one-year anniversary of the passage of the Affordable Care Act, Planned Parenthood released a statement celebrating the "important healthcare benefits and patient protections for women and families" in the act.[13] However, the press release also included details about the most recent attacks on women's reproductive rights, including significant efforts by U.S. legislators to restrict women's access to safe and legal abortion. The press release concludes on a battle-ready note: "As part of its continued support of the Affordable Care Act and women's access to comprehensive, affordable health care, Planned Parenthood will continue to fight any efforts to limit women's reproductive rights and care." While Planned Parenthood and women's health activists can advocate for women's reproductive rights (and women's health more broadly) in feminist blogs, newsletters, and other publications and through conversations with and lobbying of lawmakers, we cannot ignore the potential importance of mainstream media outlets.

Of course disrupting hegemonic media messages about women's health will be no easy task. In our current era of media deregulation and consolidation, strategies of disruption may have to originate with the audience or in the realm of public journalism, as Mary Douglas Vavrus suggests. Certainly, critical readings of public discourse about women's health like those I have offered in this project point to the need for a media literacy that questions not only what is represented in public discourse but also what is missing.[14] Part of the strength of postfeminist and neoliberal depictions of women's health is their very commonsense nature; left unquestioned, the traditional gender roles and limited methods of empowerment supported in postfeminist narratives of women's health are naturalized. The necessity of denaturalizing such depictions, whether by offering up new narratives in public discourse or through other means, is clear when we consider the material inequalities that craft women's relationships to biomedicine, their health, and their bodies. Reemphasizing a (new) feminist perspective on women's health is, I believe, an essential part of challenging the current corporatized and apolitical framing of women's health and moving in the direction of securing health for all, not merely health for a privileged few.

Notes

Introduction

1. "Go Red for Women," American Heart Association, accessed August 1, 2009, http://www.goredforwomen.org.
2. Roni Rabin, "Health Disparities Persist for Men, and Doctors Ask Why," *New York Times*, November 14, 2006.
3. Sue V. Rosser, "An Overview of Women's Health in the U.S. since the Mid-1960s," *History and Technology*18 (2002): 335.
4. "Go Red for Women: About the Movement," American Heart Association, accessed August 1, 2009, http://www.goredforwomen.org/about_the_movement.aspx.
5. Anne K. Eckman, "Beyond 'The Yentl Syndrome': Making Women Visible in Post-1990 Women's Health Discourse," in *The Visible Woman: Imaging Technologies, Gender, and Science*, edited by Paula A. Treichler, Lisa Cartwright, and Constance Penley (New York: New York University Press, 1998), 151–153; Sandra Morgen, *Into Our Own Hands: The Women's Health Movement in the United States, 1969–1990* (New Brunswick: Rutgers University Press, 2002), xi.
6. Paula Treichler uses the concept of an epidemic of signification to study public discourse about HIV/AIDS. Paula Treichler, *How to Have Theory in an Epidemic: Cultural Chronicles of AIDS* (Durham: Duke University Press, 1999).
7. Adele E. Clarke and Virginia L. Olesen, "Revising, Diffracting, Acting," in *Revisioning Women, Health, and Healing*, edited by Adele E. Clarke and Virginia L. Olesen (New York: Routledge, 1999), 9.
8. Stuart Hall, "The Toad in the Garden: Thatcherism among the Theorists," in *Marxism and the Interpretation of Culture*, edited by Cary Nelson and Larry Grossberg (Urbana: University of Illinois Press, 1988), 44.
9. Nancy Fraser, "Structuralism or Pragmatics? On Discourse Theory and Feminist Politics," in *Second Wave: A Reader in Feminist Theory*, edited by Linda J. Nicholson (New York: Routledge, 1997), 381.
10. Michel Foucault, *Power/Knowledge*, edited by Colin Gordon (New York: Pantheon Books, 1980), 131.
11. Bonnie J. Dow, *Prime-Time Feminism: Television, Media Culture, and the Women's Movement Since 1970* (Philadelphia: University of Pennsylvania Press, 1996), 7.
12. Juanne Nancarrow Clarke, "Prostate Cancer's Hegemonic Masculinity in Select Print Mass Media Depictions (1974–1995)," *Health Communication* 11 (1999): 59–74.
13. Walter Fisher, "Narration as a Human Communication Paradigm: The Case of Public Moral Argument," *Communication Monographs* 51 (1984): 6.
14. Kenneth Burke, *The Philosophy of Literary Form: Studies in Symbolic Action* (Baton Rouge: Louisiana State University Press, 1967), 293–304.
15. I understand discourse to be constitutive following the logic of Louis Althusser's theory of interpellation. All individuals live in ideology—what Althusser defines as the representation of the imaginary relationships of individuals to their real conditions of existence—and thus individuals are never without ideology, or outside of ideology. Althusser explains that "ideology 'acts' or 'functions' in such a way that it 'recruits' subjects among the individuals (it recruits them all), or 'transforms' the

individuals into subjects (it transforms them all)" through the process of interpella-tion. See Louis Althusser, "Ideology and Ideological State Apparatuses," in *Critical Theory Since 1965*, edited by Hazard Adams and Leroy Searle (Tallahassee: Florida State University Press, 1986), 245.

16. Maurice Charland, "Constitutive Rhetoric: The Case of the Peuple Quebecois," *Quarterly Journal of Speech* 73 (1987): 138.

17. See, for example, the discussion of the many factors that influence women's deci-sions about prophylactic mastectomies in Nancy Press, Susan Reynolds, Linda Pin-sky, Vinaya Murthy, Michael Leo, and Wylie Burke, "'That's Like Chopping off a Finger Because You're Afraid It Might Get Broken': Disease and Illness in Wom-en's Views of Prophylactic Mastectomy," *Social Science and Medicine* 61 (2005): 1106–1117.

18. Robert Entman, "Framing: Toward Clarification of a Fractured Paradigm," *Journal of Communication* 43 (1993): 53.

19. Susan Cheever, "What's a Memoir Writer to Do?" *Writer* 119 (2006): 20–23.

20. Judy Segal, "Breast Cancer Narratives as Public Rhetoric: Genre Itself and the Main-tenance of Ignorance," *Linguistics and the Human Sciences* 3 (2007): 16.

21. Nancy Tomes, "Patient Empowerment and the Dilemmas of Late-Modern Medicali-sation," *The Lancet* 369 (2007): 698–700.

22. Andrea L. Press and Elizabeth R. Cole, *Speaking of Abortion: Television and Author-ity in the Lives of Women* (Chicago: University of Chicago Press, 1999), 3, emphasis in original.

23. For a good analysis that compares the mainstream coverage to more targeted cover-age (in magazines aimed at African American women) of a health issue that includes representations of women of color, see Shelly Campo and Teresa Mastin, "Placing the Burden on the Individual: Overweight and Obesity in African American and Mainstream Women's Magazines," *Health Communication* 22 (2007): 229–240.

24. Michael Halliday, *Explorations in the Function of Language* (London: Edward Arnold, 1973), 22. As quoted in Barbara Barnett, "Perfect Mother or Artist of Obscen-ity? Narrative and Myth in a Qualitative Analysis of Press Coverage of the Andrea Yates Murders," *Journal of Communication Inquiry* 29 (2005): 9–29.

25. Ronald Bishop, "It's Not Always about the Money: Using Narrative Analysis to Explore Newspaper Coverage of the Act of Collecting," *The Communication Review* 6 (2003): 20; Sonja Foss, *Rhetorical Criticism: Exploration and Practice* (Prospect Heights, Ill.: Waveland Press), 400.

26. Dow, *Prime Time Feminism*, 3.

27. "Go Red for Women."

28. Ann Robertson, "Embodying Risk, Embodying Political Rationality: Women's Accounts of Risks for Breast Cancer," *Health, Risk & Society* 2 (2000): 230.

29. Tania Modleski, *Feminism without Women: Culture and Criticism in a Postfeminist Age* (London: Routledge, 1999), 49.

1. Theorizing Postfeminist Health

1. Adele E. Clarke, Laura Mamo, Jennifer R. Fishman, Janet K. Shim, and Jennifer Ruth Fosket, "Biomedicalization: Technoscientific Transformations of Health, Illness, and U.S. Biomedicine," *American Sociological Review* 68 (2003): 163.

2. Adele E. Clarke and Janet Shim, "Medicalization and Biomedicalization Revisited: Technoscience and Transformations of Health, Illness, and American Medicine," in

Handbook of the Sociology of Health, Illness, and Healing, edited by Bernice A. Pescosolido, Jack K. Martin, Jane D. McLeod, and Anne Rogers (New York: Springer, 2010), 179.

3. Ibid., 180.

4. Clarke et al., "Biomedicalization," 181; Clarke and Shim, "Medicalization," 180.

5. Nikolas Rose, "Beyond Medicalisation," *The Lancet* 369 (2007): 700.

6. Ibid.

7. Steven Epstein, *Inclusion: The Politics of Difference in Medical Research* (Chicago: University of Chicago Press, 2007), 30.

8. Ibid.

9. Ibid., 35.

10. Barbara Ehrenreich and Deidre English, *For Her Own Good: 150 Years of the Experts' Advice to Women* (New York: Anchor Books, 1978).

11. Epstein, *Inclusion*, 56.

12. Andrea O'Reilly, *Feminist Mothering* (New York: SUNY Press, 2008), 8.

13. Morgen, *Into Our Own Hands*, x.

14. Rose Kushner, *Breast Cancer: A Personal History and Investigative Report* (New York: Harcourt, Brace, Jovanovich, 1975); Barbara Seaman, *The Doctor's Case Against the Pill* (New York: Peter H. Wyden, 1969); Jennifer Nelson, "'All This That Has Happened to Me Shouldn't Happen to Nobody Else': Loretta Ross and the Women of Color Reproductive Freedom Movement of the 1980s," *Journal of Women's History* 22 (2010): 136–160; Jennifer Nelson, "'Hold Your Head up and Stick out Your Chin': Community Health and Women's Health in Mound Bayou, Mississippi," *National Women's Studies Association Journal* 17 (2005): 99–118.

15. Morgen, *Into Our Own Hands*, 4.

16. Ibid., 16–35.

17. Jael Silliman, Marlene Gerber Fried, Loretta Ross, and Elena R. Gutierrez, *Undivided Rights: Women of Color Organize for Reproductive Justice* (Cambridge, Mass.: South End Press, 2004), 55.

18. Nancy Tuana, "The Speculum of Ignorance: The Women's Health Movement and Epistemologies of Ignorance," *Hypatia* 21 (2006): 1–2.

19. Ibid., 9.

20. Anne Koedt, "The Myth of the Vaginal Orgasm," in *Radical Feminism*, edited by Anne Koedt, Ellen Levine, and Anita Rapone (New York: Quadrangle, 1973), 198–207.

21. Michelle Murphy, "Immodest Witnessing: The Epistemology of Vaginal Self-Examination in the U.S. Feminist Self-Help Movement," *Feminist Studies* 30 (2004): 118.

22. Nelson, "All This That Has Happened to Me," 139.

23. Ibid., 145.

24. Toine Largo-Janssen, "Sex, Gender & Health: Developments in Research," *European Journal of Women's Studies* 17 (2007): 10.

25. Kushner, *Breast Cancer*.

26. Toni Cade, "The Pill: Genocide or Liberation?" in *Radical Feminism: A Documentary Reader*, edited by Barbara A. Crow (New York: New York University Press, 2000), 383.

27. Ibid., 386, my emphasis.

28. Largo-Janssen, "Sex, Gender & Health," 10.

29. Morgen, *Into Our Own Hands*, 20.

30. Nelson, "All This That Has Happened to Me," 151.
31. Epstein, *Inclusion*, 56.
32. Eckman, "Beyond 'The Yentl Syndrome,'" 138.
33. Greenland and Gulati, "Improving Outcomes for Women with Myocardial Infarction," 1163.
34. Eckman, "Beyond 'The Yentl Syndrome,'" 131.
35. Ibid. 135.
36. Eckman, "Beyond 'The Yentl Syndrome,'" 133.
37. Ibid., 148.
38. Ibid., 152.
39. Epstein, *Inclusion*, 56–57.
40. Ibid., 55.
41. Ibid., 1–5.
42. Ibid., 6.
43. Ibid., 11.
44. Clarke et al., "Biomedicalization," 181.
45. Eckman, "Beyond 'The Yentl Syndrome,'" 145.
46. The literature on postfeminism is vast, but the following works are most pertinent to my research: Angela McRobbie, *The Aftermath of Feminism: Gender, Culture and Social Change* (Los Angeles: Sage, 2009); Judith Stacey, "Sexism by a Subtler Name? Postindustrial Conditions and Postfeminist Consciousness in the Silicon Valley," in *Gendered Domains*, edited by Susan Reverby and Dorothy Helly (Ithaca: Cornell University Press, 1993), 322–338; Mary Douglas Vavrus, *Postfeminist News: Political Women in Media Culture* (New York: SUNY Press, 2002); and Mary Douglas Vavrus, "Opting Out Moms in the News," *Feminist Media Studies* 7 (2007): 47–63.
47. Yvonne Tasker and Diane Negra, "Introduction: Feminist Politics and Postfeminist Culture," in *Interrogating Postfeminism: Gender and the Politics of Popular Culture*, edited by Yvonne Tasker and Diane Negra (Durham: Duke University Press, 2007), 2.
48. Rosalind Gill, "Postfeminist Media Culture: Elements of a Sensibility," *European Journal of Cultural Studies* 10 (2007): 149.
49. Nikolas Rose, *Inventing Our Selves: Psychology, Power and Personhood* (Cambridge: Cambridge University Press, 1996), 17.
50. Gill, "Postfeminist Media Culture," 154.
51. Joanne Baker, "Young Mothers in Late Modernity: Sacrifice, Respectability, and the Transformative Neoliberal Subject," *Journal of Youth Studies* 12 (2009): 277.
52. McRobbie, *The Aftermath of Feminism*, 61.
53. Ibid., 58.
54. Ibid., 64.
55. Ibid., 18.
56. Ibid., 63.
57. Joseph R. Antos, "Symptomatic Relief, but No Cure—The Obama Health Care Reform," *New England Journal of Medicine* 359 (2008): 1648.
58. Pooya S. D. Naderi and Brian D. Meier, "Privatization within the Dutch Context: A Comparison of the Health Insurance Systems of the Netherlands and the United States," *Health* 14 (2010): 606.
59. Mitchell Dean, "Risk, Calculable and Incalculable," in *Risk and Sociocultural Theory: New Directions and Perspectives*, edited by Deborah Lupton (Cambridge: Cambridge University Press, 1999), 131.
60. Ibid., 142.

61. "The Epidemic of Childhood Obesity," Let's Move, accessed June 15, 2011, http://www.letsmove.gov/learn-facts/epidemic-childhood-obesity.

62. Alan Peterson and Deborah Lupton, *The New Public Health: Health and Self in the Age of Risk* (London: Sage, 1996), 73.

63. Ibid.

64. Ibid., 79.

65. Deborah Lupton, "Risk and the Ontology of Pregnant Embodiment," in *Risk and Sociocultural Theory: New Directions and Perspectives*, edited by Deborah Lupton (Cambridge: Cambridge University Press, 1999), 60.

66. Ibid., 63.

67. Ibid., 69.

68. Ibid., 66.

69. Kelly Hannah-Moffat and Pat O'Malley, "Gendered Risks: An Introduction," in *Gendered Risks*, edited by Kelly Hannah-Moffat and Pat O'Malley (New York: Routledge-Cavendish, 2007), 20–21.

70. Ibid., 21.

71. Jessica Polzer and Ann Robertson, "From Familial Disease to 'Genetic Risk': Harnessing Women's Labour in the (Co)Production of Scientific Knowledge about Breast Cancer," in *Gendered Risks*, edited by Kelly Hannah-Moffat and Pat O'Malley (New York: Routledge-Cavendish, 2007), 33.

72. Ibid.

73. Robertson, "Embodying Risk," 230–231.

74. Hannah-Moffat and O'Malley, "Gendered Risks," 1.

75. Leo R. Chavez, F. Allen Hubbell, Juliet M. McMullin, Rebecca G. Martinez, and Shiraz I. Mishra, "Structure and Meaning in Models of Breast and Cervical Cancer Risk Factors: A Comparison of Perceptions among Latinas, Anglo Women, and Physicians," *Medical Anthropology Quarterly* 9 (1995): 69.

2. Genetic Risk

1. Bill Saporito, "He Won His Battle with Cancer. So Why are Millions of Americans Still Losing Theirs?" *Time*, September 15, 2008, 36.

2. Sharon Begley, "We Fought Cancer and Cancer Won," *Newsweek*, September 15, 2008, 42–66.

3. Ellen Leopold, *A Darker Ribbon: Breast Cancer, Women, and Their Doctors in the Twentieth Century* (Boston: Beacon Press, 1999), 20.

4. Julie Andsager and Angela Powers, "Framing Women's Wealth with a Sense-Making Approach: Magazine Coverage of Breast Cancer and Implants," *Health Communication* 13 (2001): 180.

5. See, for example, Lynn C. Hartmann, Daniel J. Schaid, John E. Woods, Thomas P. Crotty, Jeffrey L. Myers, P. G. Arnold et al., "Efficacy of Bilateral Prophylactic Mastectomy in Women with a Family History of Breast Cancer," *New England Journal of Medicine* 340 (1999): 77–84.

6. Deborah Lupton, "Femininity, Responsibility, and the Technological Imperative," *International Journal of Health Services* 24 (1994): 73.

7. Frederick Hoffman, "The Menace of Cancer," address to the American Gynecological Society, 1913. Quoted in Leopold, *A Darker Ribbon*, 155.

8. Maren Klawiter, *The Biopolitics of Breast Cancer: Changing Cultures of Disease and Activism* (Minneapolis: University of Minnesota Press, 2008), 64–65.

9. Kirsten E. Gardner, *Early Detection: Women, Cancer & Awareness Campaigns in the Twentieth-Century United States* (Chapel Hill: University of North Carolina Press, 2006), 131.

10. Klawiter, *The Biopolitics of Breast Cancer*, 84.

11. Ibid., 87.

12. Clarke et al., "Biomedicalization," 181.

13. Verta Taylor, *Rock-a-by Baby: Feminism, Self-Help and Postpartum Depression* (London: Routledge, 1996).

14. Klawiter, *The Biopolitics of Breast Cancer*, 127.

15. Sheryl Burt Ruzek and Julie Becker, "The Women's Health Movement in the United States: From Grass-Roots Activism to Professional Agendas," *Journal of the American Medical Women's Association* 54 (1999): 6; Klawiter, *The Biopolitics of Breast Cancer*, xxiii.

16. The Susan G. Komen Breast Cancer Foundation changed its name to Susan G. Komen for the Cure in 2007.

17. Nikolas Rose, "Will Biomedicine Transform Society? The Political, Economic, Social, and Personal Impact of Medical Advances in the Twenty-First Century," BIOS Working Papers. December 2008, http://www.crassh.cam.ac.uk/uploads/gallery/events/1311/rose-n.pdf, 4

18. Samantha King, *Pink Ribbons, Inc.: Breast Cancer and the Politics of Philanthropy* (Minneapolis: University of Minnesota Press, 2006), xvii.

19. Barron H. Lerner, "Inventing a Curable Disease: Historical Perspectives on Breast Cancer," in *Breast Cancer: Society Shapes an Epidemic*, edited by Anne S. Kasper and Susan J. Ferguson (New York: St. Martin's Press, 2000), 30; King, *Pink Ribbons*, xix.

20. Lerner, "Inventing a Curable Disease," 45.

21. Jennifer Ruth Fosket, "Breast Cancer Risk as Disease: Biomedicalizing Risk," in *Biomedicalization: Technoscience, Health, and Illness in the U.S.*, edited by Adele E. Clarke, Janet K. Shim, Laura Mamo, Jennifer Ruth Fosket, and Jennifer R. Fishman (Durham, N.C.: Duke University Press, 2010), 336.

22. Gina Kolata, "Panel Urges Mammograms at 50, not 40," *New York Times*, November 16, 2009.

23. Roni Rabin, "Doctor-Patient Divide on Mammograms," *New York Times*, February 15, 2010.

24. "Can Breast Cancer Be Found Early?" American Cancer Society, accessed May 1, 2011, http://www.cancer.org/Cancer/BreastCancer/DetailedGuide/breast-cancer-detection.

25. Klawiter, *The Biopolitics of Breast Cancer*, 260.

26. Peterson and Lupton, *The New Public Health*, ix.

27. Klawiter, *The Biopolitics of Breast Cancer*, 262.

28. Ibid.

29. Nikolas Rose, *The Politics of Life Itself: Biomedicine, Power, and Subjectivity in the Twenty-First Century* (Princeton, N.J.: Princeton University Press, 2006), 86.

30. Fosket, "Breast Cancer Risk as Disease," 334.

31. "Breast Cancer," American Cancer Society, accessed August 9, 2009, http://www.cancer.org/docroot/lrn/lrn_0.asp; "What Is Prevention?" National Cancer Institute, accessed May 1, 2011, http://www.cancer.gov/cancertopics/pdq/prevention/breast/Patient.

32. "Facts for Life: Breast Cancer Risk Factors," Susan G. Komen Breast Cancer Risk Factors, accessed May 1, 2011, http://ww5.komen.org/uploadedFiles/Content_Binaries/806–372a.pdf.

33. "Understanding Risk," Susan G. Komen Breast Cancer Risk Factors, accessed May 1, 2011, http://ww5.komen.org/BreastCancer/UnderstandingRisk.html.

34. "What Is Prevention?"

35. "Breast Cancer."

36. Fosket, "Breast Cancer Risk as Disease," 334.

37. "Breast Cancer."

38. Fosket, "Breast Cancer Risk as Disease," 335.

39. "Understanding Risk."

40. Rose, *The Politics of Life Itself*, 26.

41. Ibid.

42. "Breast Cancer."

43. "What Is Prevention?"

44. "Family History and Genetic Risk," Susan G. Komen Breast Cancer Foundation, accessed May 1, 2011, http://ww5.komen.org/BreastCancer/FamilyGenetics.html; Klawiter, *The Biopolitics of Breast Cancer*, 262.

45. "Inherited Genetic Mutations," Susan G. Komen Breast Cancer Foundation, accessed May 1, 2011, http://ww5.komen.org/BreastCancer/InheritedGeneticMutations.html.

46. Alan E. Guttmacher and Francis S. Collins, "Welcome to the Genomic Era," *New England Journal of Medicine* 349 (2003): 996–998.

47. Rose, *The Politics of Life Itself*, 107.

48. Ibid.

49. Ibid., 86.

50. Elisabeth Beck-Gernsheim, "Health and Responsibility: From Social Change to Technological Change and Vice Versa," in *The Risk Society and Beyond: Critical Issues for Social Theory*, edited by Barbara Adam, Ulrich Beck, and Joost Van Loon (London: Sage, 2000), 129.

51. "Cancer Previvors," FORCE web site, http://www.facingourrisk.org/info_research/previvors-survivors/cancer-previvors/index.php, accessed June 13, 2011.

52. Roni Rabin, "Study Finds Rise in Choice of Double Mastectomies," *New York Times*, October 23, 2007.

53. "Can Breast Cancer Be Prevented?" American Cancer Society, accessed May 1, 2011,http://www.cancer.org/Cancer/BreastCancer/OverviewGuide/breast-cancer-overview-prevention.

54. Fosket, "Breast Cancer Risk as Disease," 338.

55. Ibid.

56. "What Does All of This Mean For You?" American Cancer Society, accessed May 1, 2011, http://www.cancer.org/Cancer/BreastCancer/MoreInformation/Medicinesto ReduceBreastCancer/medicines-to-reduce-breast-cancer-risk-what-this-means -to-you.

57. Fosket, "Breast Cancer Risk as Disease," 339.

58. Ibid.

59. William C. Wood, "Editorial: More Answers about Prophylactic Mastectomy," *Annals of Surgical Oncology* 14 (2007): 3238.

60. Rabin, "Study Finds Rise in Choice of Double Mastectomies"; Kathleen Doheny, "More Women Choosing Preventive Double Mastectomy," *ABC News*, October

27, 2007, http://abcnews.go.com/Health/Healthday/story?id=4509131&page=1#
.TxxWXW8gpXU.

61. Hartmann et al., "Efficacy of Bilateral Prophylactic Mastectomy."
62. "Preventive Surgery," Susan G. Komen Breast Cancer Foundation, accessed May 1, 2011, http://ww5.komen.org/BreastCancer/PreventiveSurgery.html.
63. Ibid.
64. Karen Springen, "No Guarantees," *Newsweek* (web exclusive), August 27, 2008, http://www.newsweek.com/id/155864/output/print; Yu Chen, Wendy Thompson, Robert Semenciew, and Yang Mao, "Epidemiology of Contralateral Breast Cancer," *Cancer Epidemiology, Biomarkers & Prevention* 8 (1999): 855–861.
65. Derrick J. Hoover, Prakash R. Paragi, Elissa Santoro, Sarah Schafer, and Ronald S. Chamberlain, "Prophylactic Mastectomy in High Risk Patients: A Practice-Based Review of the Indications," *Breast Disease* 31 (2010): 19–27.
66. Marlene H. Frost, "Bilateral Prophylactic Mastectomy: Efficacy, Satisfaction, and Psychosocial Function," *SoCRA SOURCE* (November 2003): 30–33; Hanne Meijers-Heijboer, Cecile T. M. Brekelmans, Marian Menke-Pluymers, Caroline Seynaeve, Astrid Baalbergen, Curt Burger, Ellen Crepin, Ans W. M. van den Ouweland, Bert van Geel, and Jan G. M. Klijn, "Use of Genetic Testing and Prophylactic Mastectomy and Oophorectomy in Women with Breast or Ovarian Cancer from Families with a BRCA1 or BRCA2 Mutation," *Journal of Clinical Oncology* 21 (2003): 1675–1681.
67. Amy Harmon, "Cancer Free at 33, but Weighing a Mastectomy," *New York Times*, September 16, 2007.
68. Ibid.
69. Ibid.
70. Jessica Queller, *Pretty Is What Changes: Impossible Choices, the Breast Cancer Gene, and How I Defied My Destiny* (New York: Speigel & Grau, 2008), 7.
71. Ibid., 81.
72. Ibid., 85.
73. Ibid., 83.
74. Ibid., 85.
75. Klawiter, *The Biopolitics of Breast Cancer*, 103.
76. Queller, *Pretty Is What Changes*, 92.
77. Masha Gessen, *Blood Matters: From Inherited Illness to Designer Babies, How the World and I Found Ourselves in the Future of the Gene* (Orlando: Harcourt, Inc., 2008), 74.
78. Ibid., 130.
79. Ibid., 105.
80. Ibid., 205.
81. Steven McElroy, "Christina Applegate Battling Cancer," *New York Times*, August, 4, 2008.
82. "Christina Applegate Fighting Cancer," *ABC News*, accessed September 3, 2008, http://abcnews.go.com/print?id=5504219.
83. Christina Applegate, interview by Robin Roberts, *Good Morning America*, ABC, August 19, 2008.
84. "Christina Applegate: Why She Had a Double Mastectomy," an episode of *Oprah Winfrey Show*, first broadcast September 30, 2008, on ABC.
85. Cheryl Koopman, Lisa D. Butler, Catherine Classen, Janine Giese-Davis, Gary R. Morrow, Joan Westendorf, Tarit Banerjee, and David Spiegel, "Traumatic Stress Symptoms

among Women with Recently Diagnosed Primary Breast Cancer," *Journal of Traumatic Stress* 15 (2002): 278.

86. Gessen, *Blood Matters*, 112.
87. Christina Applegate, interview by Robin Roberts.
88. Ibid.
89. Ibid.
90. Ibid.
91. Ibid.
92. Queller, *Pretty Is What Changes*, 79.
93. Ibid., 165.
94. Ibid., 78.
95. Quoted in Queller, *Pretty Is What Changes*, 170.
96. Christina Applegate, interview by Robin Roberts; "Christina Applegate: Why She Had a Double Mastectomy."
97. Christina Applegate, interview by Robin Roberts.
98. "Christina Applegate: Why She Had a Double Mastectomy."
99. Christina Applegate, interview by Robin Roberts.
100. Beth Brophy, "Mastectomy before Breast Cancer: One Woman's Choice," *U.S. News and World Report*, April 1, 2008, http://www.usnews.com/health/managing-your -healthcare/cancer/articles/2008/04/01/mastectomy-before-breast-cancer-one -womans-choice.html.
101. Queller, *Pretty Is What Changes*, 165.
102. Ibid., 148.
103. Ibid., 238.
104. Dawn MacKeen, "Taking the Reins on 'Gossip' and Cancer," *Los Angeles Times*, May 3, 2008.
105. Susan K. Cashen, letter to the editor, *New York Times*, September 23, 2007.
106. Jennie Yabroff, "The Deepest Cut," *Newsweek* (web exclusive), April 14, 2008, http://www.newsweek.com/id/131985.
107. Deborah Lupton, introduction to *Risk and Sociocultural Theory: New Directions and Perspectives*, edited by Deborah Lupton (Cambridge: Cambridge University Press, 1999), 4.
108. Peterson and Lupton, *The New Public Health*, 49.
109. Springen, "No Guarantees."
110. Nirenejca, letter to the editor, *USA Today*, September 6, 2008, http://www.usatoday .com/news/health/2008–0819-applegate-mastectomy.
111. Christina Applegate, interview by Robin Roberts.
112. Gessen, *Blood Matters*, 7.
113. Queller, *Pretty Is What Changes*, 166.
114. Ibid.
115. Tasker and Negra, "Introduction," 10.
116. Queller, *Pretty Is What Changes*, 230.
117. Ibid., 235.
118. Sarah Bernard, "Preventive Treatment," *New York Magazine*, March 30, 2008, http:// nymag.com/arts/books/features/45569/.
119. Queller, *Pretty Is What Changes*, 242.
120. Jessica Queller, interview by Renée Montagne, *Morning Edition*, National Public Radio, April 1, 2008.

121. Diana Wagman, review of Queller, *Pretty Is What Changes*, *Los Angeles Times*, April 27, 2008.

122. Henry J. Kaiser Family Foundation, "Women's Health Insurance Coverage," *Fact Sheets: Women's Health Policy Facts*, February 2007, http://www.kff.org/womenshealth/upload/6000_05.pdf.

123. Tasker and Negra, "Introduction," 12.

124. Gill, "Postfeminist Media Culture," 149.

125. "Christina Applegate: Why She Had a Double Mastectomy."

126. Ibid.

127. Brophy, "Mastectomy before Breast Cancer."

128. Queller, *Pretty Is What Changes*, 142.

129. Ibid., 113.

130. Ibid., 133.

131. Ibid., 224.

132. Ibid., 178.

133. Ibid., 185.

134. Christina Applegate, interview by Robin Roberts.

135. "Christina Applegate: Why She Had a Double Mastectomy."

136. Carl Elliot, *Better Than Well: American Medicine Meets the American Dream* (London: Norton, 2003).

137. Queller, *Pretty Is What Changes*, 110.

138. "Christina Applegate: Why She Had a Double Mastectomy."

139. See, for example, Sandra L. Bartky, *Femininity and Domination: Studies in the Phenomenology of Oppression* (New York: Routledge, 1990); Nina Hallowell, "Reconstructing the Body or Reconstructing the Woman? Perceptions of Prophylactic Mastectomy for Hereditary Breast Cancer Risk," in *Ideologies of Breast Cancer: Feminist Perspectives*, edited by Laura K. Potts (New York: Palgrave Macmillan, 2000), 174–175.

140. Jessica Queller, interview by Renee Montagne.

141. "Christina Applegate: Why She Had a Double Mastectomy."

142. Ibid.

143. "Emmy Awards 2008: The Best Dressed Stars: Christina Applegate," *People*, September 21, 2008, http://www.people.com/people/package/gallery/0,,20225335_20227776_20513955,00.html.

144. "The Ladies Pop and Shine on the Emmys Red Carpet," *Popsugar*, September 22, 2008, http://www.popsugar.com/Red-Carpet-Photos-2008-Emmy-Awards-Including-Christina-Applegate-Heidi-Klum-Lauren-Conrad-Mary-Louise-Parker-More-2053152.

145. Hallowell, "Reconstructing the Body or Reconstructing the Woman?" 164.

146. Sue Tait, "Television and the Domestication of Cosmetic Surgery," *Feminist Media Studies* 7 (2007): 120.

147. Tasker and Negra, "Introduction," 3.

148. Audre Lorde, *The Cancer Journals* (San Francisco: Aunt Lute Books, 1997), 42.

149. Queller, *Pretty Is What Changes*, 242.

150. Klawiter, *The Biopolitics of Breast Cancer*, 38.

151. Rose, *The Politics of Life Itself*, 3.

152. Ibid., 8.

153. Judith Butler, *Gender Trouble: Feminism and the Subversion of Identity* (New York: Routledge, 1999), 44.

154. Rose, "Will Biomedicine Transform Society?" 4.

155. "Gene Patenting," Breast Cancer Action, accessed June 1, 2011, http://bcaction.org/our-take-on-breast-cancer/politics-of-breast-cancer/gene-patenting/.

156. "BCA Joins Coalition to Challenge BRCA Gene Patents," Breast Cancer Action, June 21, 2009, http://bcaction.org/2009/06/21/bca-joins-coalition-to-challenge-brca-gene-patents/.

157. Dan Vorhaus, "Breaking: District Court Rules Myriad Breast Cancer Patents Invalid," *Genomics Law Report*, March 29, 2010, http://www.genomicslawreport.com/index.php/2010/03/29/breaking-district-court-rules-myriad-breast-cancer-patents-invalid/.

158. "Gene Patenting."

159. Amanda Schaffer, "Why Are Mastectomies on the Rise? The Baffling New Breast Cancer Development," *Double X*, June 17, 2009, http://www.doublex.com/section/health-science/why-are-mastectomies-rise?page=19.

160. Ibid.

3. Postfeminist Risky Mothers and Postpartum Depression

1. Adrienne Rich, *Of Woman Born: Motherhood as Experience and Institution* (1986; New York: Norton, 1995), 13.

2. Ibid.

3. Ibid., 42.

4. Ibid., 22.

5. Angela Y. Davis, "Outcast Mothers and Reproductive Surrogates: Racism and Reproductive Politics in the Nineties," in *American Feminist Thought at Century's End: A Reader*, edited by Linda S. Kauffman (Cambridge, Mass.: Blackwell, 1993), 355.

6. Roderick Hart, *Modern Rhetorical Criticism*, 2nd ed. (Boston: Allyn & Beacon, 1997), 234.

7. Susan Douglas and Meredith Michaels, *The Mommy Myth: The Idealization of Motherhood and How It Has Undermined Women* (New York: Free Press, 2004), 20.

8. Lauri Umansky, *Motherhood Reconceived: Feminism and the Legacy of the Sixties* (New York: New York University Press, 1996), 4.

9. Ibid., 123, 140.

10. Barnett, "Perfect Mother or Artist of Obscenity?"; Barbara Barnett, "Medea in the Media: Narrative and Myth in Newspaper Coverage of Women Who Kill Their Children," *Journalism* 7 (2006): 411–432.

11. My goal when reviewing blogs was to read and analyze blogs that had the most cultural capital (blogs that were read by a good number of people, blogs that were referred to by other blogs, and so forth). I began my search with Babble.com's top 50 "Mommy Blogs": http://www.babble.com/babble-50/mommy-bloggers/. (Their number-two blogger is Heather Armstrong.) I also included in my analysis blogs that ranked highly (in the top 50) at topmommyblogs.com.

12. Verta Taylor, *Rock-a-by Baby: Feminism, Self-Help, and Postpartum Depression* (New York: Routledge, 1996), 2.

13. Ibid.

14. Ibid.

15. Ibid., 2–8.

16. Linda M. Blum and Nena F. Stracuzzi, "Gender in the Prozac Nation: Popular Discourse and Productive Femininity," *Gender & Society* 18 (2004): 271.

17. Ibid.

18. Rose, *The Politics of Life Itself*, 194.

19. Laura J. Miller, "Postpartum Depression," *Journal of the American Medical Association* 287 (2002): 762.

20. Michael W. O'Hara, "Postpartum Depression: What We Know," *Journal of Clinical Psychology* 65 (2009): 1258.

21. Ibid., 1259.

22. Ibid.

23. Susan Hatters Friedman, "Postpartum Mood Disorders: Genetic Progress and Treatment Paradigms," *American Journal of Psychiatry* 166 (2009): 1201.

24. Uriel Halbreich, "Women's Reproductive Related Disorders (RRDs)," *Journal of Affective Disorders* 122 (2010): 11.

25. Ibid., 11–12.

26. Anne Fausto-Sterling, *Myths of Gender: Biological Theories about Women and Men* (New York: Basic Books, 1995), 90–122.

27. Rose, *The Politics of Life Itself*, 199.

28. Paula Nicolson, "Postpartum Depression: Women's Accounts of Loss and Change," in *Situating Sadness: Women and Depression in Social Context*, edited by Janet M. Stoppard and Linda M. McMullen (New York: New York University Press, 2003), 119.

29. Laura Brown, "Discomforts of the Powerless: Feminist Constructions of Distress," in *Constructions of Disorder: Meaning Making Frameworks for Psychotherapy*, edited by Robert A. Neimeyer and Jonathan D. Raskin (Washington, D.C.: American Psychological Association, 2000), 287.

30. Taylor, *Rock-a-by Baby*, 6.

31. Ibid., 70.

32. Ibid., 40–46.

33. Brown, "Discomforts of the Powerless," 287.

34. Rose, "Beyond Medicalisation," 701.

35. Umansky, *Motherhood Reconceived*, 76.

36. Rose, "Beyond Medicalisation," 701.

37. Taylor, *Rock-a-by Baby*, 158.

38. Renee Martinez, Ingrid Johnston-Robledo, Heather M. Ulsh, and Joan C. Chrisler, "Singing 'the Baby Blues'": A Content Analysis of Popular Press Articles about Postpartum Affective Disturbances," *Women & Health* 31 (2000): 51.

39. Ibid.

40. David Hochman, "Mommy (And Me)," *New York Times*, January 30, 2005.

41. Kate Arosteguy, "The Politics of Race, Class, and Sexuality in Contemporary American Mommy Lit," *Women's Studies* 39 (2010): 411.

42. Lisa Belkin, "Let the Kids Be," *New York Times*, May 31, 2009.

43. "About," A Bad Mommy's Blog, accessed July 30, 2010, http://abadmommyblog.wordpress.com/huh/.

44. "Real Moms," A Bad Mommy's Blog, accessed July 30, 2010, http://abadmommyblog.wordpress.com/real-moms/.

45. Heather Armstrong, *It Sucked and Then I Cried: How I Had a Baby, a Breakdown, and a Much Needed Margarita* (New York: Gallery Books, 2009), 214.

46. "Oxygen Mask," *Pretty All True* (blog), July 14, 2010, http://www.prettyalltrue.com/2010/07/oxygen-mask/.

47. Ibid.

48. Susan, "About Me," Domestic Diva blog, accessed July 30, 2010, http://www.divine secretsofadomesticdiva.com/about/.

49. Ibid.

50. Mrs. Foreste, "Work, Work, Work," As the Forest(e) Grows blog, July 9, 2010, http://mrsforeste.blogspot.com/2010/07/work-work-work.html.

51. Sarah, "The Greatest Love," Becoming Sarah blog, July 12, 2010, http://becomingsarah.com/index.php?/becoming_sarah/comments/975/.

52. Brooke Shields, *Down Came the Rain: My Journey through Postpartum Depression* (New York: Hyperion, 2005), 189.

53. Catherine Connors, Her Bad Mother blog, accessed July 30, 2010,http://herbad mother.com.

54. Catherine Connors, "The Bad Mother Manifesto," Her Bad Mother blog, June 8, 2009, http://herbadmother.com/2009/06/bad-mother-manifesto/.

55. See, for example, Mary Douglas Vavrus, "Opting Out Moms in the News: Selling New Traditionalism in the New Millennium," *Feminist Media Studies* 7 (2007): 47–63.

56. Jeni Harden argues that risks regarding children, like all other risks, are "constructed" (that is, we focus selectively on certain risks over others). Although public discourse often focuses on risks to children outside the home, the fear of "stranger danger" overshadows the very real risks children encounter at home. In the United States, the discourse of "new momism" has focused on mothers in relation to many of the risks children encounter at home. The current emphasis on breastfeeding accepts the notion that women place their children at risk if they bottle feed. The rise in educational toys—and the drive to buy them—is also premised on risk: mothers who do not purchase the right toys put their child's intellectual development at risk. See Jeni Harden, "There's No Place Like Home: The Public/Private Distinction in Children's Theorizing of Risk and Safety," *Childhood* 7 (2000): 43–44; Douglas and Michaels, *The Mommy Myth*, 292–295.

57. Catherine Connors, "10 Things I Hate about Motherhood and 1 That I Love," Her Bad Mother blog, April 20, 2010, http://herbadmother.com/2010/04/10-things -i-hate-about-motherhood-and-one-that-i-love/.

58. Connors, "The Bad Mother Manifesto."

59. Vavrus, *Postfeminist News*, 25.

60. Jane E. Brody, "Don't Let Your Baby Blues Go Code Red," *New York Times*, June 7, 2005.

61. Shields, *Down Came the Rain*, 74.

62. Ibid., 70.

63. Armstrong, *It Sucked and Then I Cried*, 168.

64. Ibid., 123.

65. Ibid., 124.

66. Stefanie Wilder-Taylor, "Worry, the Circular Emotion," Baby on Bored blog, March 14, 2009, http://stefaniewildertaylor.com/2009/03/worry-circular-emotion/.

67. Katie, "Frustration," Cleared for Takeoff: The (Un)Glamorous Life of a Pilot's Wife blog, July 1, 2010, http://www.takeoffwithkatie.com/2010/07/frustration.html.

68. Kimberly, "The Beginning of My Descent," All Work and No Play Make Mommy Go Something Something (blog), November 3, 2009, http://makemommygosomething something.wordpress.com/2009/11/03/the-begining-of-my-decent/.

69. The most famous drinking "bad mommy" is Stefanie Wilder Taylor, author of *Sippy Cups Are Not for Chardonnay* and *Naptime Is the New Happy Hour*. See also Jan

Hoffman, "A Heroine of Cocktail Moms Sobers Up," *New York Times*, August 16, 2009.

70. Katherine Stone, "The Unrelenting Self-Doubt and Second-Guessing of Postpartum Depression & Anxiety," Postpartum Progress blog, February 8, 2010, http://postpartumprogress.typepad.com/weblog/2010/02/the-unrelenting-selfdoubt-and-secondguessing-of-postpartum-depression-anxiety.html.

71. Brooke Shields, "War of Words," *New York Times*, July 1, 2005.

72. Susan Gilbert, "Estrogen Patch Appears to Lift Severe Depression in New Mothers," *New York Times*, May 1, 1996.

73. Shields, "War of Words."

74. Ibid.

75. Katherine Stone, "6 Things Every New Mom Should Know about Postpartum Depression," *Postpartum Progress* (blog), accessed July 30, 2010, http://postpartumprogress.typepad.com/.

76. Armstrong, *It Sucked and Then I Cried*, 252.

77. Ibid., 3.

78. Davi A. Johnson, "Managing Mr. Monk: Control and the Politics of Madness," *Critical Studies in Media Communication* 25 (2008): 28–47.

79. Shields, *Down Came the Rain*, 144.

80. Gwyneth Paltrow, "Be," *Goop Newsletter*, July 22, 2010, http://goop.com/newsletter/93/en/.

81. Alice Park, "Postpartum Depression Strikes New Fathers Too," *Time*, May 18, 2010, http://www.time.com/time/health/article/0,8599,1989805,00.html.

82. Barbara Ehrenreich, "Welcome to Cancerland: A Mammogram Leads to a Cult of Pink Kitsch," *Harper's Magazine*, November 2001, 49.

83. Although Nikolas Rose suggests that the process of (bio)medicalization does not individualize (that is, focus on the self as problem and solution) because it actually creates "new ways of tracing connections and making connections" among individuals and groups, in this case individualization is an important aspect of public discourse about postpartum depression. See Rose, "Will Biomedicine Transform Society?" 9.

84. Johnson, "Managing," 32.

85. Shields, *Down Came the Rain*, 223.

86. Johnson, "Managing Mr. Monk," 32.

87. Ibid., 42.

88. "Gwyneth's Guide to Life," *Vogue*, May 2008, 258.

89. Johnson, "Managing Mr. Monk," 33.

90. Armstrong, *It Sucked and Then I Cried*, 122.

91. Ibid.

92. Ibid., 169.

93. Ibid., 190.

94. Kimberly, "Bad Days Will Happen," All Work and No Play Make Mommy Go Something Something blog, November 9, 2009, http://makemommygosomethingsomething.wordpress.com/2009/11/09/bad-days-will-happen/.

95. Julie, "Postpartum Anxiety: Caused by the Baby or Caused by the Act of Parenting?" Postpartum Progress blog, July 15, 2010, http://www.postpartumprogress.com/weblog/2010/07/postpartum-anxiety-caused-by-the-baby-or-the-act-of-parenting.html.

96. Paula Span, "Making Sure Mothers Start on the Right Foot," *New York Times*, April 9, 2006.

97. Shields, *Down Came the Rain*, 115, emphasis in original.

98. Ibid., 116.

99. Ibid., 164.

100. Ibid., 165.

101. Ibid., 167.

102. Katherine Stone, "5 Things Dads Can Do to Understand & Help with Postpartum Depression," ThisEmotionalLifeblog, December 7, 2009, http://www.pbs.org/thisemotionallife/blogs/5-things-dads-can-do-understand-help-postpartum-depression.

103. Women such as Heather Armstrong who experience severe anxiety during the postpartum period are often diagnosed with and refer to themselves as having postpartum depression. My use of "postpartum depression" thus encompasses women who are treated with antidepressants for anxiety and obsessive-compulsive symptoms.

104. Shields, *Down Came the Rain*, 83.

105. Ibid., 142.

106. Lisa M. Cuklanz and Sujata Moorti, "Television's 'New' Feminism: Prime Time Representations of Women and Victimization," *Critical Studies in Media Communication* 23 (2006): 314.

107. Katherine Stone, "ABC Television Should be ASHAMED of 'Private Practice' Postpartum Psychosis Treatment," Postpartum Progress blog, February 13, 2009, http://www.postpartumprogress.com/weblog/2009/02/abc-television-should-be-ashamed-of-private-practice-postpartum-psychosis-treatment.html.

108. Tasha N. Dubriwny, "Television News Coverage of Postpartum Disorders and the Politics of Medicalization," *Feminist Media Studies* 10 (2010): 285–303.

109. Shields, *Down Came the Rain*, 71.

110. Lauren Hale, "Graham Crackers and Peanut Butter Served with a Side of Crazy: Part 1," My Postpartum Voice blog, May 31, 2010, http://mypostpartumvoice.com/2010/05/31/graham-crackers-and-peanut-butter-part-i/.

111. Lauren Hale, "Graham Crackers and Peanut Butter Served with a Side of Crazy: Part 3," My Postpartum Voice blog, June 2, 2010, http://mypostpartumvoice.com/2010/06/02/graham-crackers-peanut-butter-with-a-side-order-of-crazy-part-iii/.

112. "Woman Not Guilty in Retrial In the Deaths of Her 5 Children," *New York Times*, July 27, 2006.

113. Richard Weir, "Names, Dignity and Hope: Dumped, Dead Newborns Get TLC from Foundation," *New York Daily News*, March 4, 2007.

114. Ibid.

115. Associated Press, "Dead Baby's Father Says Mother Should Be Executed," *Long Island Press*, July 28, 2009, http://www.longislandpress.com/2009/07/28/dead-babys-father-says-mother-should-be-executed/.

116. Ann Berryman, Deborah Fowler, Hilary Hylton, and Greg Fulton, "The Yates Odyssey," *Time*, July 26, 2006, http://www.time.com/time/magazine/article/0,9171,1001706-1,00.html.

117. Ibid.

118. Ibid.

119. Ibid.

120. Ibid.

121. Dirk Johnson and Carol Rust, "'Who's Babysitting the Kids?'" *Newsweek*, January 17, 2005, 37.

122. Shields, *Down Came the Rain*, 114.
123. Katherine Stone, "An Open Letter to Time Magazine about Postpartum Depression," Postpartum Progress blog, July 14, 2009, http://postpartumprogress.com/open-letter -to-time-magazine-about-postpartum-depression.
124. Ibid.
125. Rose, "Beyond Medicalisation," 702.
126. Shields, *Down Came the Rain*, 136.
127. Drew Humphries, *Crack Mothers: Pregnancy, Drugs, and the Media* (Columbus: Ohio State University Press, 1999), 11.
128. Ibid.
129. Dubriwny, "Television News Coverage of Postpartum Disorders."
130. Jayne Huckerby, "Women Who Kill Their Children: Case Study and Conclusions Concerning the Differences in the Fall from Maternal Grace by Khoua Her and Andrea Yates," *Duke Journal of Gender Law & Policy* 10 (2003): 166.
131. Taylor, *Rock-a-by Baby*, 179.
132. Ibid., 162.
133. Roni Rabin, "Having a Baby: Depression Affects New Fathers, Too," *New York Times*, May 25, 2010.
134. Ibid.
135. Liz Szabo, "New Dads Hit by Depression as Often as Moms," *USA Today*, May 19, 2010.
136. Liz Szabo, "Dad's Pregnancy Hormones," *USA Today*, June 15, 2010.
137. Ibid.
138. Joel Schwartzberg, "Slouching toward Fatherhood," *Newsweek*, April 13, 2009, 17.
139. "Postpartum Depression in Men?" *The Week*, May 19, 2010, http://theweek.com/ article/index/203133/postpartum-depression-in-men.
140. Park, "Postpartum Depression Strikes New Fathers, Too."
141. Rosemary Black, "Dads Can Get Postpartum Depression, Too," *Daily News*, May 19, 2010, http://www.nydailynews.com/lifestyle/health/2010/05/19/2010–05–19 _dads_can_get_postpartum_depression_too_study.html.
142. Lisa Belkin, "Postpartum Depression and Fathers," *New York Times*, August 14, 2009, http://parenting.blogs.nytimes.com/2009/08/14/colic-postpartum-depression -and-fathers/.
143. Laurie Tarkan, "After the Adoption, a New Child and the Blues," *New York Times*, April 25, 2006.
144. Ibid.

4. The Postfeminist Concession

1. Stephanie Saul and Andrew Pollack, "Furor on Rush to Require Vaccine," *New York Times*, February 17, 2007; "Preventing Cancer or Promoting Sex?" *Dallas Morning News*, February 10, 2007.
2. Shobha S. Krishnan, *The HPV Vaccine Controversy. Sex, Cancer, God, and Politics: A Guide for Parents, Women, Men, and Teenagers* (Westport, Conn.: Praeger, 2008), 65–69.
3. Monica J. Casper and Laura M. Carpenter, "Sex, Drugs, and Politics: The HPV Vaccine for Cervical Cancer," *Sociology of Health & Illness* 30 (2008): 892.
4. Karen Houppert, "Who's Afraid of Gardasil?" *The Nation*, March 26, 2007, http:// www.thenation.com/article/whos-afraid-gardasil.

5. Yvonne Collins, Mark H. Einstein, Bobbie S. Gostout, Thomas J. Herzog, L. Stewart Massad, Janet S. Rader, and Jason Wright, "Cervical Cancer Prevention in the Era of Prophylactic Vaccines: A Preview for Gynecologic Oncologists," *Gynecologic Oncology* 102 (2006): 553.

6. Eliav Barr and Heather L. Sings, "Prophylactic HPV Vaccines: New Interventions for Cancer Control," *Vaccine* 26 (2008): 6245.

7. Collins et al., "Cervical Cancer," 553.

8. Ibid.

9. Krishnan, *The HPV Vaccine Controversy*, 66.

10. Rose, "Will Biomedicine Transform Society?" 5.

11. Chandra Talpade Mohanty, "Feminism without Borders," in *Feminist Frontiers*, 8th ed., edited by Verta Taylor, Nancy Whittier, and Leila J. Rupp (Boston: McGraw-Hill, 2009), 97.

12. Laura M. Carpenter and Monica J. Casper, "Global Intimacies: Innovating the HPV Vaccine for Women's Health," *Women's Studies Quarterly* 37 (2009): 88.

13. Ibid.

14. Ibid., 80.

15. Ibid., 87.

16. Ibid., 89.

17. Ibid., 82.

18. Ibid., 91.

19. Ibid.

20. Donald G. McNeil Jr., "How a Vaccine Search Ended in Triumph," *New York Times*, August 29, 2006.

21. Valerie Beral, "Cancer of the Cervix: A Sexually Transmitted Infection?" *The Lancet* 303 (1974): 1037–1040.

22. McNeil, "How a Vaccine Search Ended in Triumph."

23. Virginia Braun and Nicola Gavey, "'Bad Girls' and 'Good Girls'? Sexuality and Cervical Cancer," *Women's Studies International Forum* 22 (1999): 205.

24. Casper and Carpenter, "Sex, Drugs, and Politics," 888.

25. Adina Nack, "Bad Girls and Fallen Women: Chronic STD Diagnoses as Gateways to Tribal Stigma," *Symbolic Interaction* 25 (2002): 465.

26. Braun and Gavey, "'Bad Girls' and 'Good Girls,'" 204.

27. "Protection with Gardasil," *Gardasil*, accessed May 1, 2010, http://www.gardasil .com/what-is-gardasil/cervical-cancer-vaccine/index.html.

28. Marie Thompson, "Who's Guarding What? A Poststructural Feminist Analysis of Gardasil Discourses," *Health Communication* 25 (2010): 119.

29. Ibid., 122.

30. Ibid., 122.

31. Ibid., 123.

32. Casper and Carpenter, "Sex, Drugs, and Politics," 886; Paula Treichler, *How to Have Theory in an Epidemic: Cultural Chronicles of AIDS* (Durham, N.C.: Duke University Press, 1999), 43.

33. Treichler, *How to Have Theory*, 43.

34. Judith Siers-Poisson, "Research, Develop, and Sell, Sell, Sell: Part Two in a Series on the Politics and PR of Cervical Cancer," *PRWatch*, June 30, 2007, http://prwatch.org/ node/6208.

35. Beth Herskovits, "Brand of the Year," *Pharmaceutical Executive*, February 1, 2007, http://pharmexec.findpharma.com/pharmexec/Articles/Brand-of-the-Year/ArticleStandard/Article/detail/401664.

36. Kelley J. Main, Jennifer J. Argo, and Bruce A. Huhmann, "Pharmaceutical Advertising in the USA: Information or Influence?" *International Journal of Advertising* 23 (2004): 121.

37. I focus primarily on two advertisements that aired nationally in 2007 and portions of the web site geared toward supplementing the televised "One Less" commercials. One of these advertisements is currently available on YouTube. References to the second advertisement are from my handwritten notes from 2007. To access the previous iterations of the Gardasil.com web site, I used the Wayback Machine Internet search engine.

38. "Gardasil Commercial [A]," November 13, 2006, YouTube video, http://www.youtube.com/watch?v=hJ8x3KR75fA&feature=related, accessed May 1, 2010.

39. Bree Kessler and Summer Wood, "A Shot in the Dark: What—and Who—Is Behind the Marketing of Gardasil?" *Bitch Magazine*, Summer 2007, 27–32.

40. Sumi Cho, "Post-Racialism," *Iowa Law Review* 94–95 (2009): 1594.

41. Kent A. Ono, "Postracism: A Theory of the 'Post-' as Political Strategy," *Journal of Communication Inquiry* 34 (2010): 227–233.

42. Lisa Traiger, "Stomp the Stage: Tradition Meets Contemporary Rhythm at Step Afrika's Spirited Performance," *Dance Magazine*, February 2009, 40–42.

43. "Gardasil Commercial [A]."

44. Ibid.

45. "Double Dutch: Fun and Great Exercise," The African American Registry web site, accessed May 1, 2010,http://www.aaregistry.org/historic_events/view/double-dutch-fun-and-great-exercise.

46. Kessler and Wood, "A Shot in the Dark."

47. Claire Dederer, "Pitching Protection, to Both Mothers and Daughters," *New York Times*, February 18, 2007.

48. "Gardasil Commercial [A]."

49. "Gardasil," Gardasil web site, December 3, 2006, http://www.gardasil.com. Accessed May 1, 2010 through the Wayback Machine Internet Archive, http://www.archive.org/web/web.php.

50. Although I am referring here to the 2006–2007 version of the web site, the avoidance of the term "sexually transmitted" continues in more recent iterations of the site.

51. "Gardasil Commercial [A]."

52. Marnina Gonick, "Between 'Girl Power' and 'Reviving Ophelia': Constituting the Neoliberal Girl Subject," *National Women's Studies Association Journal* 18 (2006): 2.

53. Ibid., 6.

54. Ibid., 10.

55. "Gardasil Commercial [A]."

56. Ibid.

57. Casper and Carpenter, "Sex, Drugs, and Politics," 893.

58. Ibid.

59. Angela Zimm and Justin Blum, "Merck Promotes Cervical Cancer Shot by Publicizing Viral Cause," Bloomberg, May 26, 2006, http://www.bloomberg.com/apps/news?pid=newsarchive&sid=amVj.y3Eynz8&refer=us.

60. Ibid.

61. Allison L. Friedman and Hilda Shepeard, "Exploring the Knowledge, Attitudes, Beliefs, and Communication Preferences of the General Public Regarding HPV: Findings from CDC Focus Group Research and Implications for Practice," *Health Education and Behavior* 34 (2007): 473.

62. Ibid., 478.

63. David J. Rothman and Sheila M. Rothman, "Marketing HPV Vaccine: Implications for Adolescent Health and Medical Professionalism," *Journal of the American Medical Association* 302 (2009): 782.

64. Ibid.

65. Jessica Polzer and S. Knabe, "Good Girls Do . . . Get Vaccinated: HPV, Mass Marketing and Moral Dilemmas for Sexually Active Young Women," *Journal of Epidemiology and Community Health* 63 (2009): 869.

66. Thomas P. Boyle, "Intermedia Agenda Setting in the 1996 Presidential Election," *Journalism & Mass Communication Quarterly* 28 (2001): 26.

67. To my knowledge, no research has been done on the ability of direct-to-consumer advertisements to "set the agenda" for the understanding of a particular drug. However, such studies have been done in the political sphere. As Boyle reports, one study found a "strong correlation between television political advertising, and television news and newspaper coverage"; ibid., 28. Many studies indicate the influence of direct-to-consumer advertisements on consumer choice and doctor/patient conversations. See, for example, Angela Hausman, "Direct-to-Consumer Advertising and Its Effect on Prescription Requests," *Journal of Advertising Research* 48 (2008): 42–56.

68. Kathy Davis, "Paternalism under the Microscope," in *Gender and Discourse: The Power of Talk*, edited by A. Todd and S. Fisher (Norwood, N.J.: Ablex, 1988), 23.

69. Paul Achter, Kevin Kuswa, and Elizabeth Lauzon, "The Slave, the Fetus, the Body: Articulating Biopower and the Pregnant Woman," *Contemporary Argumentation and Debate* 29 (2008): 174.

70. Reva B. Siegel, "Dignity and the Politics of Protection: Abortion Restrictions under *Casey/Carhart*," *Yale Law Journal* 1694 (2008): 1776.

71. Corrie MacLaggan, "Perry Requires HPV Vaccine for Girls," *Austin-American Statesman*, February 3, 2007.

72. Ibid.

73. Alberta Phillips, "Furor Shows That What's Right Isn't Always Popular," *Austin-American Statesman*, February 26, 2007.

74. Casper and Carpenter, "Sex, Drugs and Politics, and Politics," 888; Kessler and Wood, "A Shot in the Dark," 32; Lynn Weber and Deborah Parra-Medina, "Intersectionality and Women's Health: Charting a Path to Eliminating Health Disparities," *Advances in Gender Research* 7 (2003): 184.

75. For a larger explanation of relational inequalities, see Weber and Parra-Medina, "Intersectionality and Women's Health," 217.

76. Gloria Steinem, "Supremacy Crimes," *Ms. Magazine*, August 1999, 45.

77. Suzanne M. Horn, letter to the editor, *Houston Chronicle*, February 12, 2007.

78. James Nelson, letter to the editor, *Austin American-Statesman*, February 9, 2007.

79. Penna Dexter, "First Person: Protecting Our Girls," *Baptist Press News*, January 18, 2007, http://www.bpnews.net/bpnews.asp?id=24796.

80. Jacquielynn Floyd, "HPV Vaccine Is a Lifesaver Tossed Aside," *Dallas Morning News*, March 2, 2007.

81. Rick Perry, "Remarks on the Decision Regarding House Bill 1098," May 8, 2007, http://governor.state.tx.us/news/speech/5525/.

82. Ibid.

83. Phyllis Marynick Palmer, "White Women/Black Women: The Dualism of Female Identity and Experience in the United States," *Feminist Studies* 9 (1983): 156.

84. Adrienne Rich, "Compulsory Heterosexuality and Lesbian Existence," in *The Lesbian and Gay Studies Reader*, edited by Henry Abelove, Michele Aina Barale, and David M. Halperin (New York: Routledge, 1993), 228, 238.

85. Corrie MacLaggan, "Perry's HPV Vaccine Order Draws Backlash from GOP," *Austin-American Statesman*, February 6, 2007.

86. Corrie MacLaggan, "Perry Bows to Vaccine Order's Foes," *Austin-American Statesman*, May 9, 2007.

87. Corrie MacLaggan, "A Push to Start HPV Shots This Fall," *Austin-American Statesman*, February 13, 2007.

88. Phillips, "Furor Shows That What's Right Isn't Always Popular."

89. Gardiner Harris, "U.S. Approves Use of Vaccine for Cervical Cancer," *New York Times*, June 9, 2006.

90. Harris, "U.S. Approves Use of Vaccine."

91. Perry, "Remarks on the Decision Regarding House Bill 1098."

92. Ibid.

93. "Heather Burcham on the HPV Vaccine," May 8, 2007, YouTube video, http://www .youtube.com/watch?v=OIsWB348z-Q, accessed May 1, 2010.

94. Ralph Blumenthal, "Texas Is First to Require Cancer Shots for Schoolgirls," *New York Times*, February 3, 2007.

95. Jessica Farrar and Raymond H Kaufman, "Arm Young Texans with the Facts on HPV," *Austin-American Statesman*, February 15, 2007.

96. Alan Katz, letter to the editor, *New York Times*, February 10, 2007.

97. Barbara Adam and Joost van Loon, "Introduction: Repositioning Risk; the Challenge for Social Theory," in *The Risk Society and Beyond: Critical Issues for Social Theory*, edited by Barbara Adam, Ulrich Beck, and Joost van Loon (London: Sage, 2000), 4.

98. Elizabeth Beiter Milford, letter to the editor, *New York Times*, February 10, 2007.

99. Sarah Beshers, "Abstinence-What? A Critical Look at the Language of Educational Approaches to Adolescent Sexual Risk Reduction," *Journal of School Health* 77 (2007): 638.

100. Jessica Fields, "'Children Having Children': Race, Innocence, and Sexuality Education," *Social Problems* 52 (2005): 549–571.

101. Quoted in Gardiner Harris, "Panel Unanimously Recommends Cervical Cancer Vaccine for Girls 11 and Up," *New York Times*, June 30, 2006.

102. Fields, "'Children Having Children,'" 560.

103. Deborah L. Tolman, *Dilemmas of Desire: Teenage Girls Talk about Sexuality* (Cambridge, Mass.: Harvard University Press, 2002), 171.

104. MacLaggan, "Perry Requires HPV Vaccine for Girls."

105. MacLaggan, "Perry's HPV Vaccine Order Draws Backlash."

106. Ann Friedman, "Our Best Shot," The American Prospect web site, February 1, 2007, http://www.prospect.org/cs/articles?articleId=12428.

107. Tolman, *Dilemmas of Desire*, 1–24.

108. Jane E. Brody, "HPV Vaccine: Few Risks, Many Benefits," *New York Times*, May 15, 2007.

109. Corrie MacLaggan, "Health Panel Gets Testimony on Vaccine," *Austin-American Statesman*, February 20, 2007.

110. Rick Perry, "Letter Accompanying the Announcement of the Decision Regarding HB 1098," May 8, 2007, accessed May 1, 2010, http://www.nccc-online.org/health_news/topics/controversial/rick_perry.html.

111. Denise Grady, "A Vital Discussion, Clouded," *New York Times*, March 6, 2007.

112. Perry, "Letter Accompanying the Announcement of the Decision Regarding HB 1098."

113. Peterson and Lupton, *The New Public Health*, 16.

114. Saul and Pollack, "Furor on Rush to Require Vaccine."

115. Jill Stanek, "Debbie Does . . . ??," *Illinois Review*, February 6, 2007, http://illinoisreview.typepad.com/illinoisreview/2007/02/debbie_halvorso.html.

116. Dexter, "First Person."

117. Ibid.

118. Andrew Pollack and Stephanie Saul, "Lobbying for Vaccine to Be Halted," *New York Times*, February 21, 2007.

119. "Gardasil Commercial [B]," June 6, 2008, YouTube video, http://www.youtube.com/watch?v=ZHUamYNSH9c&feature=related, accessed May 1, 2010.

120. Ibid.

121. "Gardasil TV Commercial," October 6, 2009, YouTube video, http://www.youtube.com/watch?v=15Jk30Bm31U&feature=related, accessed May 1, 2010.

122. Ibid.

123. "Merck Gardasil HPV Vaccine I Chose Ad #1," June 11, 2008, YouTube video, http://www.youtube.com/watch?v=ehvxbEOgNEM&feature=related, accessed May 1, 2010.

124. "Gardasil Commercial [B]."

125. "Gardasil TV Commercial."

126. "Merck Gardasil HPV Vaccine I Chose Ad #1."

127. Ibid.

128. Rose, "Will Biomedicine Transform Society?" 4.

129. Because my analysis focused on the construction of the "at-risk/risky young woman" and her relationship to the risk of sex, I did not focus on the growing discourse questioning the safety of Gardasil. This discourse was present even at the beginning of the controversy, with concerned parents, doctors, and health experts questioning the safety of mandating a vaccine so soon after its approval. Now that the vaccine has been on the market for several years, reports of adverse events have increased. One potential area of intervention for feminist health activists could very well be studying and/or questioning the vaccine's safety and efficacy records. That said, when I discuss the "largely unquestioning nature" of that consumption, I am referring to how the identity of the "at-risk/risky young woman"—in all spheres of discourse, including the early Gardasil campaign—does not include space for questions from adolescents and women about the safety of the vaccine.

130. The FDA approved Gardasil for the use in males ages nine to twenty-six in October 2009. "FDA Approves New Indication for Gardasil to Prevent Genital Warts in Men and Boys," *U.S. Food and Drug Administration*, October 16, 2009, http://www.fda.gov/NewsEvents/Newsroom/PressAnnouncements/ucm187003.htm.

131. Rose, *The Politics of Life Itself*, 40.

5. Feminist Women's Health Activism in the Twenty-first Century

1. Virginia L. Olesen and Adele E. Clarke, "Resisting Closure, Embracing Uncertainties, Creating Agendas," in *Revisioning Women, Health, and Healing: Feminist,*

Cultural, and Technoscience Perspectives, edited by Adele E. Clarke and Virginia L. Olesen (New York: Routledge, 1999), 356.

2. Gardiner Harris, "It Started More Than One Revolution," *New York Times*, May 30, 2010.

3. Ibid.

4. Elizabeth Kissling, "How the Pill Gave Birth to the Women's Health Movement," Ms. Blog, May 24, 2010, http://msmagazine.com/blog/blog/2010/05/24/how-the-pill-gave-birth-to-the-women%E2%80%99s-health-movement/.

5. Ibid.

6. Ibid.

7. Ruzek and Becker, "The Women's Health Movement," 4.

8. Marjorie Bowman and Marcy Lynn Gross, "Overview of Research on Women in Medicine—Issues for Public Policymakers," *Public Health Reports* 101 (1986): 514.

9. Epstein, *Inclusion*, 56.

10. Ibid., 10.

11. Ruzek and Becker, "The Women's Health Movement," 6.

12. Lisa Duggan, *The Twilight of Equality? Neoliberalism, Cultural Politics, and the Attack on Democracy* (Boston: Beacon Press, 2003), xii.

13. Ibid., xvii.

14. Ruzek and Becker, "The Women's Health Movement," 6.

15. Ibid., 6.

16. Epstein, *Inclusion*, 56.

17. Vavrus, *Postfeminist News*, 23.

18. Although I did not explore the issue here, cervical cancer screening programs using the Pap smear produced a specific understanding of femininity in which a normal part of being a woman includes regular surveillance by and interaction with the medical system. Judith Bush explains, "This study suggests that cervical screening is not just about surveillance of the cervix and women's sexuality but it also encompassed getting women to behave in a particular, prescribed way. Cervical screening is built upon medical discourses concerning the need for *regulation* of women's bodies." Specifically, an entire series of behaviors related to cervical screening—disrobing, the exposure of body parts, the acceptance of an internal examination—are normalized by the expectation that women will receive yearly pap smears. Judith Bush, "'It's Just Part of Being a Woman': Cervical Screening, the Body, and Femininity," *Social Science and Medicine* 50 (2000): 432, 441.

19. Miriam Yeung and Amanda Allen, "Immigrant Women: A Victory on the Road to Reproductive Justice," *RH Reality Check*, December 1, 2009, http://www.rhrealitycheck.org/print/12057.

20. Ibid.

21. My search for news coverage included a search of newspapers in the LexisNexis Academic database. A search for articles using the three terms "papillomavirus," "immigration," and "vaccine" over the past five years returned six articles, only two of which were in national newspapers (*USA Today* and *Wall Street Journal*). A similar search (for articles using both "HPV" and "immigration") returned one more article from a local paper in El Paso, Texas.

22. Julie Jordan, "She Is My Beginning," *People*, February 28, 2011, 60–66. The reference to this story on the cover of the magazine declares, "Christina Applegate, Baby After Breast Cancer, She Is My Miracle!"

23. "Author Takes Steps to Fight Cancer, Become Mom," *NPR Morning Edition*, June 30, 2009, http://www.npr.org/templates/story/story.php?storyId=105797044.

24. Jennifer Waite, "Christina Applegate Pregnant: New Baby by Spring 2011 for Applegate and Fiancé, Martyn Lenoble," Yahoo! Voices web site, July 22, 2010, http://www.associatedcontent.com/article/5610478/christina_applegate_pregnant_new_baby.html.

25. Rose, *The Politics of Life Itself*, 4.

26. Rosemary Hertz to National Women's Health Network, September 21, 2001, National Women's Health Network Records, 1975–1996, Box 13, Folder "Fall Appeal 2001 'Bush Watch' 9/7/01," Sophia Smith Collection, Smith College, Northampton, Massachusetts.

27. For an appealing discussion of why a "logic of care" may be a better approach to health than our current "logic of choice," see Annemarie Mol, *The Logic of Care: Health and the Problem of Patient Choice* (London: Routledge, 2008).

28. Phaedra Pezzullo, "Resisting 'National Breast Cancer Awareness Month': The Rhetoric of Counterpublics and Their Cultural Performances," *Quarterly Journal of Speech* 89 (2003): 345–365.

29. Ibid., 351.

30. Rose, *The Politics of Life Itself*, 105.

31. Laura Mamo, "Fertility, Inc.," in *Biomedicalization: Technoscience, Health, and Illness in the U.S.*, edited by Adele E. Clarke, Janet K. Shim, Laura Mamo, Jennifer Ruth Fosket, and Jennifer R. Fishman (Durham, N.C.: Duke University Press, 2010), 177.

32. Rose, "Will Biomedicine Transform Society?" 8.

33. Ibid. See also Paul Rabinow, *Essays on the Anthropology of Reason* (Princeton, N.J.: Princeton University Press, 1996), 91–111.

34. Rose, *The Politics of Life Itself*, 95.

35. Ibid., 128.

36. Ibid., 129.

37. Sahra Gibbon and Carlos Novas, "Introduction: Biosocialities, Genetics and the Social Sciences," *Biosocialities, Genetics, and the Social Sciences: Making Biologies and Identities*, edited by Sahra Gibbon and Carlos Novas (London: Routledge, 2008), 2.

38. "History and Victories," Breast Cancer Action web site, accessed June 13, 2011, http://bcaction.org/about/history-victories/.

39. Rose, *The Politics of Life Itself*, 140–141.

40. Ibid., 144.

41. Ibid., 174.

42. "History and Victories."

43. Ibid.

44. "Breast Cancer Action's Screening Recommendations," Breast Cancer Action web site, accessed June 13, 2011, http://bcaction.org/policy-on-breast-cancer-screening-and-early-detection/.

45. Olesen and Clarke, "Resisting Closure," 356.

46. Adele E. Clarke, Janet K. Shim, Laura Mamo, Jennifer Ruth Fosket, and Jennifer R. Fishman, "Biomedicalization: A Theoretical and Substantive Introduction," in *Biomedicalization: Technoscience, Health, and Illness in the U.S.*, edited by Adele E. Clarke, Janet K. Shim, Laura Mamo, Jennifer Ruth Fosket, and Jennifer R. Fishman (Durham, N.C.: Duke University Press, 2010), 14.

47. "Aromatase Inhibitors," Breast Cancer Action web site, accessed June 13, 2011, http://bcaction.org/our-take-on-breast-cancer/treatment/aromatase-inhibitors/.

48. "Our Priorities," Breast Cancer Action web site, accessed June 13, 2011, http://bcaction.org/about/priorities/.

49. "Think Before You Pink," Think Before You Pink web site, accessed June 1, 2010, http://thinkbeforeyoupink.org/.

50. Jennifer Myhre, "The Breast Cancer Movement: Seeing beyond Consumer Activism," *Journal of the American Medical Women's Association* 54 (1999): 29.

51. "Yoplait: Put a Lid on It," Think Before You Pink web site, accessed June 1, 2010, http://thinkbeforeyoupink.org/?page_id=10.

52. "Clean Cars," Think Before You Pink web site, accessed June 1, 2010, http://think beforeyoupink.org/?page_id=17.

53. Pezzullo, "Resisting 'National Breast Cancer Awareness Month,'" 358.

54. "Our Priorities."

55. "Cancer Previvors," FORCE web site, accessed June 13, 2011, http://www.facingour risk.org/info_research/previvors-survivors/cancer-previvors/index.php.

56. Rita M. Bair, Rose M. Mays, Lynne A. Sturm, and Gregory D. Zimet, "Acceptability of the Human Papillomavirus Vaccine among Latina Mothers," *Journal of Pediatric Adolescent Gynecology* 21 (2008): 329.

57. Weber and Parra-Medina, "Intersectionality and Women's Health," 181.

58. Melissa A. Thomasson, "From Sickness to Health: The Twentieth-Century Development of U.S. Health Insurance," *Explorations in Economic History* 39 (2002): 233.

59. Jonathan Cohn, *Sick: The Untold Story of America's Health Care Crisis—and the People Who Pay the Price* (New York: HarperCollins, 2007), 6.

60. Jacob S. Hacker and Theda Skocpol, "The New Politics of U.S. Health Policy," *Journal of Health Politics, Policy and Law* 22 (1997): 321; Cohn, *Sick*.

61. Cohn, *Sick*, 9.

62. Ibid., 10.

63. Ibid., 21.

64. Antos, "Symptomatic Relief, but No Cure," 1648.

65. Uwe E. Reinhardt, Peter S. Hussey, and Gerard F. Anderson, "U.S. Health Care Spending in an International Context," *Health Affairs* 23 (2004): 12.

66. Hacker and Skocpol, "The New Politics of U.S. Health Policy," 323–324.

67. See, for example, Paul Krugman, "Runaway Health Costs—We're #1!" *New York Times*, March 28, 2008, http://krugman.blogs.nytimes.com/2008/03/28/runaway -health-care-costs-were-1/.

68. Barbara Starfield, "Is US Health Really the Best in the World?" *Journal of the American Medical Association* 284 (2000): 483.

69. Ibid.

70. Ibid., 484–485.

71. "Topics: Health Care Reform," *New York Times*, March 4, 2011, http://topics .nytimes.com/top/news/health/diseasesconditionsandhealthtopics/health_insurance _and_managed_care/health_care_reform/index.html.

72. David U. Himmelstein and Steffie Woolhandler, "Obama's Reform: No Cure for What Ails Us," *British Medical Journal* 340 (2010): 742.

73. Epstein, *Inclusion*, 125.

74. Ibid., 74.

75. Ibid., 298.

76. Ibid., 297.

77. Ibid., 299.

78. Weber and Parra-Medina, "Intersectionality and Women's Health," 183–184.

79. National Association of Social Workers, "Reproductive Health Disparities for Women of Color," December 2004, http://www.socialworkers.org/diversity/Equity1204.pdf.

80. Celeste Condit Railsback, "The Contemporary American Abortion Controversy: Stages in the Argument," [1984], in *Readings on the Rhetoric of Social Protest*, 2nd ed., edited by Charles E. Morris III and Stephen Howard Browne (State College, Pa.: Strata Publishing, 2006), 478.

81. Ibid.

82. The Hyde Amendment is a rider that has been attached to congressional appropriations bills every year since 1976. The amendment bans federal Medicaid funding of abortions in almost all circumstances.

83. Andrea Smith, "Beyond Pro-Choice Versus Pro-Life: Women of Color and Reproductive Justice," *Feminist Formations* 17 (2005): 129.

84. Ibid., 130.

85. Sara Hayden, "Revitalizing the Debate Between <Life> and <Choice>: The 2004 March for Women's Lives," *Communication and Critical/Cultural Studies* 6 (2009): 112.

86. Ibid., 121.

87. Ibid.

88. Ibid., 122.

89. John W. Delicath and Kevin Michael DeLuca, "Image Events, the Public Sphere, and Argumentative Practice: The Case of Radical Environmental Groups," *Argumentation* 17 (2003): 330; Hayden, "Revitalizing the Debate," 128.

90. Morgen, *Into Our Own Hands*, 41–42.

91. Ibid., 53.

92. Weber and Parra-Medina, "Intersectionality and Women's Health," 194.

93. Loretta Ross to SisterSong Conference participants, undated e-mail, National Women's Health Network Records, 1975–1996, Box 14, Folder "March for Choice," Sophia Smith Collection, Smith College, Northampton, Massachusetts.

94. SisterSong, "A Solidarity Statement from SisterSong Women of Color Reproductive Health Collective October 2003," National Women's Health Network Records,1975–1996 Box 14, Folder "March for Choice," Sophia Smith Collection, Smith College, Northampton, Massachusetts.

95. Lynn Roberts, "March to Save Women's Lives," *Collective Voices* 1, no. 2 (2003): 4.

96. Eveline Shen, "Asian Communities for Reproductive Justice Answers the Question: What Is Reproductive Justice?" *Collective Voices* 1, no. 2 (2004): 6.

97. Ibid.

98. Weber and Parra-Medina, "Intersectionality and Women's Health," 187.

99. Ibid.

100. Ibid., 188.

101. Ibid., 222.

102. Peter Osborne and Lynn Segal, "Gender as Performance: An Interview with Judith Butler," *Radical Philosophy* 67 (1994): 32–39.

103. Epstein, *Inclusion*, 248.

104. Ibid., 253.

105. Hannah-Moffat and O'Malley, "Gendered Risks," 5.

106. Ibid., 3.

107. Ibid., 5.

108. "Scarleteen Is," Scarleteen web site, accessed June 1, 2010, http://www.scarleteen
.com/scarleteen_is.

109. Heather Corinna, "What Is Feminist Sex Education?" Scarleteen web site, accessed
June 1, 2010, http://www.scarleteen.com/article/politics/what_is_feminist_sex
_education.

110. Weber and Parra-Medina, "Intersectionality and Women's Health," 193.

111. Heather Corinna, "20 Questions about Virginity: Scarleteen Interviews Hanne
Blank," Scarleteen web site, accessed June 1, 2010, http://www.scarleteen.com/
article/politics/20_questions_about_virginity_scarleteen_interviews_hanne_blank.

112. Ibid.

113. "About Scarleteen," Scarleteen web site, accessed June 1, 2010, http://www.scarleteen
.com/about_scarleteen.

114. Ibid.

115. Ibid.

116. For an excellent overview and critique of liberal understandings of autonomy, see
Anne Phillips, "Feminism and Liberalism Revisited: Has Martha Nussbaum Got It
Right?" *Constellations* 8 (2001): 249–266.

117. Clarke and Olesen, "Revising, Diffracting, Acting," 4.

118. Polzer and Robertson, "From Familial Disease to 'Genetic Risk,'" 48.

119. James Darsey, "From 'Gay Is Good' to the Scourge of AIDS: The Evolution of Gay
Liberation Rhetoric," [1991], in *Readings on the Rhetoric of Social Protest*, 2nd ed.,
edited by Charles E. Morris III and Stephen Howard Browne (State College, Pa.:
Strata Publishing, 2006), 500.

120. Clarke and Olesen, "Revising, Diffracting, Acting," 10.

121. "The STI Files: Human Papillomavirus," Scarleteen web site, accessed June 1, 2010,
http://www.scarleteen.com/article/infection/the_sti_files_human_papillomavirus
_hpv.

122. Heather Corinna, "I Guess You Just Have to Be Prepared to Die," Scarleteen web site,
October 31, 2009, http://www.scarleteen.com/blog/heather_corinna/2009/10/31/
i_guess_you_just_have_to_be_prepared_to_die.

123. Ibid.

124. Ibid.

125. "Eli Lilly and rBGH," Think Before You Pink web site, accessed June 1, 2010, http://
thinkbeforeyoupink.org/?page_id=2.

126. "Building the Future," Breast Cancer Action web site, accessed May 1, 2011, http://
archive.bcaction.org/index.php?page=bca-s-plan.

127. Ester Shapiro, "Because Words Are Not Enough: Latina Re-Visionings of Trans-
national Collaborations Using Health Promotion for Gender Justice and Social
Change," in *Diversity and Women's Health*, edited by Sue V. Rosser (Baltimore, Md.:
Johns Hopkins University Press, 2009), 65.

128. Cecilia M. B. Sardenberg, "Liberal vs. Liberating Empowerment: A Latin American
Feminist Perspective on Conceptualising Women's Empowerment," *IDS Bulletin* 39
(2008): 18.

129. "Building the Future."

Afterword

1. "Action Alert: Women's March Coverage Hard to Find on Television News," Fair-
ness and Accuracy in Reporting web site, May 3, 2004, http://www.fair.org/activism/
womens-march-networks.html.

2. Ibid.

3. "MomsRising," MomsRising.org web site, accessed February 27, 2012, http://www
.momsrising.org.

4. "M: Maternity Leave," MomsRising.org web site, accessed June 30, 2010, http://
www.momsrising.org/page/moms/maternity.

5. Adina Nack, "Why Men's Health Is a Feminist Issue," *Ms. Magazine*, Winter 2010,
http://www.msmagazine.com/winter2010/menshealth.asp; Amanda Hess, "The
Feminist Implications of Male Reproductive Health," *Washington City Paper*, February 4, 2010, http://www.washingtoncitypaper.com/blogs/sexist/2010/02/24/the
-feminist-implications-of-male-reproductive-health/.

6. Hess, "The Feminist Implications of Male Reproductive Health."

7. Donna Shelley, "Establishing Women's Health Centers in Academic Institutions:
Obstacles and Opportunities," *Journal of the American Medical Women's Association* 54 (1999): 12, 9.

8. Stephen S. Cha, Joseph S. Ross, Peter Lurie, and Galit Sacajiu, "Description of a
Research-Based Activism Curriculum for Medical Students," *Journal of General
Internal Medicine* 21 (2006): 1325.

9. Sharon Lerner, "Medical Students Go Beyond Books to Learn about Activism," *New
York Times*, December 2, 2003.

10. "Women's Health Advocates Call for Better Healthcare Reform," Our Bodies, Our
Blog, January 20, 2010, http://www.ourbodiesourblog.org/blog/2010/01/womens
-health-advocates-call-for-better-healthcare-reform.

11. Ibid.

12. "House Votes to Strip Planned Parenthood of Federal Funding," *ABC News*, February 18, 2011, http://abcnews.go.com/Politics/house-votes-strip-planned-parenthood
-federal-funding/story?id-12951080.

13. "Planned Parenthood Commemorates Adoption of the Historic Affordable Care Act,
Highlighting the Promise of Reform and Warning of Continued Efforts to Reverse
It," *Planned Parenthood*, March 22, 2011, http://www.plannedparenthood.org/
about-us/newsroom/press-releases/planned-parenthood-commemorates-adoption
-historic-affordable-care-act-highlighting-promise-refo-36535.htm.

14. Vavrus, *Postfeminist News*, 184.

Bibliography

Achter, Paul, Kevin Kuswa, and Elizabeth Lauzon. "The Slave, the Fetus, the Body: Articulating Biopower and the Pregnant Woman." *Contemporary Argumentation and Debate* 29 (2008): 166–185.

Adam, Barbara, and Joost van Loon. "Introduction: Repositioning Risk; the Challenge for Social Theory." In *The Risk Society and Beyond: Critical Issues for Social Theory*, edited by Barbara Adam, Ulrich Beck, and Joost van Loon, 1–31. London: Sage, 2000.

Althusser, Louis. "Ideology and Ideological State Apparatuses." In *Critical Theory Since 1965*, edited by Hazard Adams and Leroy Searle, pp. 239–251. Tallahassee: Florida State University Press, 1986.

Antos, Joseph R. "Symptomatic Relief, but No Cure—the Obama Health Care Reform." *New England Journal of Medicine* 359 (2008): 1648–1650.

Andsager, Julie, and Angela Powers. "Framing Women's Health with a Sense-Making Approach: Magazine Coverage of Breast Cancer and Implants." *Health Communication* 13 (2001): 163–185.

Applegate, Christina. Interview by Robin Roberts on *Good Morning America*, ABC, broadcast August 19, 2008.

Armstrong, Heather. *It Sucked and Then I Cried: How I Had a Baby, a Breakdown, and a Much Needed Margarita*. New York: Gallery Books, 2009.

Arosteguy, Kate. "The Politics of Race, Class, and Sexuality in Contemporary American Mommy Lit." *Women's Studies* 39 (2010): 409–429.

Associated Press. "Dead Baby's Father Says Mother Should Be Executed." *Long Island Press*. July 28, 2009. At http://www.longislandpress.com/2009/07/28/dead-babys-father-says-mother-should-be-executed. Accessed January 22, 2012.

"Author Takes Steps to Fight Cancer, Become Mom." *Morning Edition*, National Public Radio, aired June 30, 2009. Transcript available at http://www.npr.org/templates/story/story.php?storyId=105797044. Accessed January 22, 2012.

Bair, Rita M., Rose M. Mays, Lynne A. Sturm, and Gregory D. Zimet. "Acceptability of the Human Papillomavirus Vaccine among Latina Mothers." *Journal of Pediatric Adolescent Gynecology* 21 (2008): 329–334.

Baker, Joanne. "Young Mothers in Late Modernity: Sacrifice, Respectability, and the Transformative Neoliberal Subject." *Journal of Youth Studies* 12 (2009): 275–288.

Barnett, Barbara. "Medea in the Media: Narrative and Myth in Newspaper Coverage of Women Who Kill Their Children." *Journalism* 7 (2006): 411–432.

———. "Perfect Mother or Artist of Obscenity? Narrative and Myth in a Qualitative Analysis of Press Coverage of the Andrea Yates Murders." *Journal of Communication Inquiry* 29 (2005): 9–29.

Barr, Eliav, and Heather L. Sings. "Prophylactic HPV Vaccines: New Interventions for Cancer Control." *Vaccine* 26 (2008): 6244–6257.

Bartky, Sandra L. *Femininity and Domination: Studies in the Phenomenology of Oppression*. New York: Routledge, 1990.

Beck-Gernsheim, Elisabeth. "Health and Responsibility: From Social Change to Technological Change and Vice Versa." In *The Risk Society and Beyond: Critical Issues for*

Social Theory, edited by Barbara Adam, Ulrich Beck, and Joost Van Loon, 122–135. London: Sage, 2000.

Begley, Sharon. "We Fought Cancer and Cancer Won." *Newsweek*, September 15, 2008, 42–66.

Belkin, Lisa. "Let the Kids Be." *New York Times*, May 31, 2009.

Beral, Valerie. "Cancer of the Cervix: A Sexually Transmitted Infection." *Lancet* 303 (1974): 1037–1040.

Bernard, Sarah. "Preventive Treatment." *New York Magazine*, March 30, 2008. At http:// nymag.com/arts/books/features/45569/. Accessed January 21, 2012.

Berryman, Ann, Deborah Fowler, Hilary Hylton, and Greg Fulton. "The Yates Odyssey." *Time*, July 26, 2006. At http://www.time.com/time/magazine/article/0,9171,1001706,00 .html. Accessed January 21, 2012.

Beshers, Sarah. "Abstinence-What? A Critical Look at the Language of Educational Approaches to Adolescent Sexual Risk Reduction." *Journal of School Health* 77 (2007): 637–669.

Bishop, Ronald. "It's Not Always about the Money: Using Narrative Analysis to Explore Newspaper Coverage of the Act of Collecting." *The Communication Review* 6 (2003): 117–135.

Black, Rosemary. "Dads Can Get Postpartum Depression, Too." *Daily News*, May 19, 2010.

Blum, Linda M., and Nena F. Stracuzzi. "Gender in the Prozac Nation: Popular Discourse and Productive Femininity." *Gender & Society* 18 (2004): 269–286.

Blumenthal, Ralph. "Texas Is First to Require Cancer Shots for Schoolgirls." *New York Times*, February 3, 2007.

Bowman, Marjorie, and Marcy Lynn Gross. "Overview of Research on Women in Medicine—Issues for Public Policymakers." *Public Health Reports* 101 (1986): 513–521.

Boyle, Thomas P. "Intermedia Agenda Setting in the 1996 Presidential Election." *Journalism & Mass Communication Quarterly* 28 (2001): 26–44.

Braun, Virginia, and Nicola Gavey. "'Bad Girls' and 'Good Girls'? Sexuality and Cervical Cancer." *Women's Studies International Forum* 22 (1999): 203–213.

Brody, Jane E. "Don't Let Your Baby Blues Go Code Red." *New York Times*, June 7, 2005.

———. "HPV Vaccine: Few Risks, Many Benefits." *New York Times*, May 15, 2007.

Brophy, Beth. "Mastectomy before Breast Cancer: One Woman's Choice." *U.S. News & World Report*, April 1, 2008. At http://www.usnews.com/health/managing-your -healthcare/cancer/articles/2008/04/01/mastectomy-before-breast-cancer-one-womans -choice.html. Accessed January 22, 2012.

Brown, Laura. "Discomforts of the Powerless: Feminist Constructions of Distress." In *Constructions of Disorder: Meaning Making Frameworks for Psychotherapy*, edited by Robert A. Neimeyer and Jonathan D. Raskin, 287–308. Washington, D.C.: American Psychological Association, 2000.

Burke, Kenneth. *The Philosophy of Literary Form: Studies in Symbolic Action*. Baton Rouge: Louisiana State University Press, 1967.

Bush, Judith. "'It's Just Part of Being a Woman': Cervical Screening, the Body, and Femininity." *Social Science and Medicine* 50 (2000): 429–444.

Butler, Judith. "Gender as Performance: An Interview with Judith Butler." By Peter Osborne and Lynn Segal. *Radical Philosophy* 67 (1994): 32–39.

———. *Gender Trouble: Feminism and the Subversion of Identity*. New York: Routledge, 1999.

Cade, Toni. "The Pill: Genocide or Liberation?" In *Radical Feminism: A Documentary Reader*, edited by Barbara A. Crowe, 382–387. New York: New York University Press, 2000.

Campo, Shelly, and Teresa Mastin. "Placing the Burden on the Individual: Overweight and Obesity in African American and Mainstream Women's Magazines." *Health Communication* 22 (2007): 229–240.

Carpenter, Laura M., and Monica J. Casper. "Global Intimacies: Innovating the HPV Vaccine for Women's Health." *Women's Studies Quarterly* 37 (2009): 80–100.

Cashen, Susan K. Letter to the Editor. *New York Times*, September 23, 2007.

Casper, Monica J., and Laura M. Carpenter. "Sex, Drugs, and Politics: The HPV Vaccine for Cervical Cancer." *Sociology of Health & Illness* 30 (2008): 886–899.

Cha, Stephen S., Joseph S. Ross., Peter Lurie, and Galit Sacajiu. "Description of a Research-Based Activism Curriculum for Medical Students." *Journal of General Internal Medicine* 21 (2006): 1325–1328.

Charland, Maurice. "Constitutive Rhetoric: the Case of the Peuple Quebecois." *Quarterly Journal of Speech* 73 (1987): 133–150.

Chavez, Leo R., F. Allan Hubbell, Juliet M. McMullin, Rebecca G. Martinez, and Shiraz I. Mishra. "Structure and Meaning in Models of Breast and Cervical Cancer Risk Factors: A Comparison of Perceptions among Latinas, Anglo Women, and Physicians." *Medical Anthropology Quarterly* 9 (1995): 40–74.

Cheever, Susan. "What's a Memoir Writer to Do?" *Writer* 119 (2006): 20–23.

Chen, Yu, Wendy Thompson, Robert Semenciew, and Yang Mao. "Epidemiology of Contralateral Breast Cancer." *Cancer Epidemiology Biomarkers & Prevention* 8 (1999): 855–861.

Cho, Sumi. "Post-Racialism." *Iowa Law Review* 94–95 (2009): 1589–1648.

Clarke, Adele E., Laura Mamo, Jennifer R. Fishman, Janet K. Shim, and Jennifer Ruth Fosket. "Biomedicalization: Technoscientific Transformations of Health, Illness, and U.S. Biomedicine." *American Sociological Review* 68 (2003): 161–194.

Clarke, Adele E., and Virginia L. Olesen. "Revising, Defracting, Acting." In *Revisioning Women, Health, and* Healing, edited by Adele L. Clarke and Virginia L. Olesen, 3–48. New York: Routledge, 1999.

Clarke, Adele E., and Janet Shim. "Medicalization and Biomedicalization Revisited: Technoscience and Transformations of Health, Illness, and American Medicine." In *Handbook of the Sociology of Health, Illness, and Healing*, edited by Bernice A. Pescosolido, Jack K. Martin, Jane D. McLeod, and Anne Rogers, 173–199. New York: Springer, 2010.

Clarke, Adele E., Janet K. Shim, Laura Mamo, Jennifer Ruth Fosket and Jennifer R. Fishman. "Biomedicalization: A Theoretical and Substantive Introduction." In *Biomedicalization: Technoscience, Health, and Illness in the U.S.*, edited by Adele E. Clarke, Janet K. Shim, Laura Mamo, Jennifer Ruth Fosket, and Jennifer R. Fishman, 1–47. Durham, N.C.: Duke University Press, 2010.

Clarke, Juanne Nancarrow. "Prostate Cancer's Hegemonic Masculinity in Select Print Mass Media Depictions (1974–1995)." *Health Communication* 11 (1999): 59–74.

Cohn, Jonathan. *Sick: The Untold Story of America's Health Care Crisis—and the People Who Pay the Price*. New York: HarperCollins, 2007.

Collins, Yvonne, Mark H. Einstein, Bobbie S. Gostout, Thomas J. Herzog, L. Stewart Massad, Janet S. Rader, and Jason Wright, "Cervical Cancer Prevention in the Era of Prophylactic Vaccines: A Preview for Gynecologic Oncologists." *Gynecologic Oncology* 102 (2006): 552–562.

Cuklanz, Lisa M. and Sujata Moorti. "Television's 'New' Feminism: Prime Time Representations of Women and Victimization." *Critical Studies in Media Communication* 23 (2006): 302–321.

Darsey, James. "From 'Gay Is Good' to the Scourge of AIDS: The Evolution of Gay Liberation Rhetoric" [1991]. In *Readings on the Rhetoric of Social Protest*, 2nd ed., edited by Charles E. Morris III and Stephen Howard Browne, 486–507. State College, Pa.: Strata Publishing, 2006.

Davis, Angela Y. "Outcast Mothers & Reproductive Surrogates: Racism and Reproductive Politics in the Nineties." In *American Feminist Thought at Century's End: A Reader*, edited by Linda S. Kaufmann, 355–366. Cambridge, Mass.: Blackwell, 1993.

Davis, Flora. *Moving the Mountain: The Women's Movement in America since 1960*. Chicago: University of Illinois Press, 1999.

Davis, Kathy. "Paternalism under the Microscope." In *Gender and Discourse: The Power of Talk*, edited by A Todd and S. Fisher, 19–54. Norwood, N.J.: Ablex, 1988.

Dean, Mitchell. "Risk, Calculable and Incalculable." In *Risk and Sociocultural Theory: New Directions and Perspectives*, edited by Deborah Lupton, 131–159. Cambridge: Cambridge University Press, 1999.

Dederer, Claire. "Pitching Protection, to Both Mothers and Daughters." *New York Times*, February 18, 2007.

Delicath, John W., and Kevin Michael DeLuca. "Image Events, the Public Sphere, and Argumentative Practice: The Case of Radical Environmental Groups." *Argumentation* 17 (2003): 315–333.

Dexter, Penna. "First Person: Protecting Our Girls." *Baptist Press News*, January 18, 2007. At http://www.bpnews.net/bpnews.asp?id=24796. Accessed January 22, 2012.

Doheny, Kathleen. "More Women Choosing 'Preventive' Double Mastectomy." *U.S. News and World Report*, October 22, 2007. http://abcnews.go.com/Health/Healthday/story?id=4509131&page=1#.TxxWXW8gpXU.

Douglas, Susan, and Meredith Michaels. *The Mommy Myth: The Idealization of Motherhood and How It Has Undermined Women*. New York: Free Press, 2004.

Dow, Bonnie J. *Prime-Time Feminism: Television, Media Culture, and the Women's Movement Since 1970*. Philadelphia: University of Pennsylvania Press, 1996.

Dubriwny, Tasha N. "Television News Coverage of Postpartum Disorders and the Politics of Medicalization." *Feminist Media Studies* 10 (2010): 285–303.

Duggan, Lisa. *The Twilight of Equality? Neoliberalism, Cultural Politics, and the Attack on Democracy*. Boston: Beacon Press, 2003.

Eckman, Anne K. "Beyond 'The Yentl Syndrome': Making Women Visible in Post-1990 Women's Health Discourse." In *The Visible Woman: Imaging Technologies, Gender, and Science*, edited by Paula A. Treichler, Lisa Cartwright, and Constance Penley, 131–168. New York: New York University Press, 1998.

Ehrenreich, Barbara. "Welcome to Cancerland: A Mammogram Leads to a Cult of Pink Kitsch." *Harper's Magazine*, November 2001, 43–53.

Ehrenreich, Barbara, and Deirdre English. *For Her Own Good: 150 Years of the Experts' Advice to Women*. New York: Anchor Books, 1978.

Elliot, Carl. *Better Than Well: American Medicine Meets the American Dream*. London: Norton, 2003.

"Emmy Awards 2008: The Best Dressed Stars: Christina Applegate." *People*, September 21, 2008. At http://www.people.com/people/package/gallery/0,,20225335_20227776_20513955,00.html. Accessed January 22, 2012.

Entman, Robert. "Framing: Toward Clarification of a Fractured Paradigm." *Journal of Communication* 43 (1993): 51–58.

Epstein, Steven. *Inclusion: the Politics of Difference in Medical Research.* Chicago: University of Chicago Press, 2007.

Farrar, Jessica, and Raymond H. Kaufman. "Arm Young Texans with the Facts on HPV." *Austin-American Statesman*, February 15, 2007.

Fausto-Sterling, Anne. *Myths of Gender: Biological Theories about Women and Men.* New York: Basic Books, 1995.

Fields, Jessica. "'Children Having Children': Race, Innocence, and Sexuality Education." *Social Problems* 52 (2005): 549–571.

Fisher, Walter. "Narration as Human Communication Paradigm: The Case of Public Moral Argument." *Communication Monographs* 51 (1984): 1–22.

Floyd, Jacquielynn. "HPV Vaccine Is a Lifesaver Tossed Aside." *Dallas Morning News*, March 2, 2007.

Fosket, Jennifer Ruth. "Breast Cancer Risk as Disease: Biomedicalizing Risk." In *Biomedicalization: Technoscience, Health, and Illness in the U.S.*, edited by Adele E. Clarke, Janet K. Shim, Laura Mamo, Jennifer Ruth Fosket, and Jennifer R. Fishman, 331–352. Durham, N.C.: Duke University Press, 2010.

Foss, Sonja. *Rhetorical Criticism: Exploration and Practice.* Prospect Heights, Ill.: Waveland Press, 1989.

Foucault, Michel. *Power/Knowledge.* Edited by Colon Gordon. New York: Pantheon Books, 1980.

Fraser, Nancy. "Structuralism or Pragmatics? On Discourse Theory and Feminist Politics." In *Second Wave: A Reader in Feminist Theory*, edited by Linda J. Nicholson, 379–395. New York: Routledge, 1997.

Friedman, Allison L., and Hilda Shepeard. "Exploring the Knowledge, Attitudes, Beliefs, and Communication Preferences of the General Public Regarding HPV: Findings from CDC Focus Group Research and Implications for Practice." *Health Education and Behavior* 34 (2007): 471–485.

Friedman, Ann. "Our Best Shot." *The American Prospect*, February 1, 2007. http://prospect.org/article/our-best-shot.

Friedman, Susan Hatters. "Postpartum Mood Disorders: Genetic Progress and Treatment Paradigms." *American Journal of Psychiatry* 166 (2009): 1201–1204.

Frost, Marlene H. "Bilateral Prophylactic Mastectomy: Efficacy, Satisfaction, and Psychosocial Function." *SoCRA SOURCE* (November 2003). At http://www.socra.org/pdf/200311_BilateralProphylacticMastectomy.pdf. Accessed January 22, 2012.

"Gardasil Commercial [A]." November 13, 2006. YouTube video. At http://www.youtube.com/watch?v=hJ8x3KR75fA&feature=related. Accessed May 1, 2010.

"Gardasil Commercial [B]." June 6, 2008. YouTube video. At http://www.youtube.com/watch?v=ZHUamYNSH9c&feature=related. Accessed May 1, 2010.

"GARDASIL TV Commercial." October 6, 2009. YouTube video. At http://www.youtube.com/watch?v=15Jk30Bm31U&feature=related. Accessed May 1, 2010.

Gardner, Kirsten E. *Early Detection: Women, Cancer, and Awareness Campaigns in the Twentieth-Century United States.* Chapel Hill: University of North Carolina Press, 2006.

Gessen, Masha. *Blood Matters: From Inherited Illness to Designer Babies, How the World and I Found Ourselves in the Future of the Gene.* Orlando, Fla.: Harcourt, Inc., 2008.

Gibbon, Sahra, and Carlos Nova. "Introduction: Biosocialities, Genetics, and the Social Sciences." In *Biosocialities, Genetics, and the Social Sciences: Making Biologies and Identities*, edited by Sahra Gibbon and Carlos Nova, 1–18. New York: Routledge, 2008.

Gilbert, Susan. "Estrogen Patch Appears to Lift Severe Depression in New Mothers." *New York Times*, May 1, 1996.

Gill, Rosalind. "Postfeminist Media Culture: Elements of a Sensibility." *European Journal of Cultural Studies* 10 (2007): 147–166.

Gonick, Marnina. "Between 'Girl Power' and 'Reviving Ophelia': Constituting the Neoliberal Girl Subject." *National Women's Studies Association Journal* 18 (2006): 1–23.

Grady, Denise. "A Vital Discussion, Clouded." *New York Times*, March 6, 2007.

Greenland, Philip, and Martha Gulati. "Improving Outcomes for Women with Myocardial Infarction." *Archives of Internal Medicine* 166 (2006): 1162–1163.

Guttmacher, Alan E., and Francis S. Collins. "Welcome to the Genomic Era." *New England Journal of Medicine* 349 (2003): 996–998.

"Gwyneth's Guide to Life." *Vogue*, May 2008, 258.

Hacker, Jacob S., and Theda Skocpol. "The New Politics of U.S. Health Policy." *Journal of Health Politics, Policy and Law* 22 (1997): 315–338.

Halbreich, Uriel. "Women's Reproductive Related Disorders (RRDs)." *Journal of Affective Disorders* 122 (2010): 10–13.

Hall, Stuart. "The Toad in the Garden: Thatcherism among the Theorists." In *Marxism and the Interpretation of Culture*, edited by Cary Nelson and Larry Grossberg, 35–74. Urbana: University of Illinois Press, 1988.

Halliday, Michael. *Explorations in the Function of Language*. London: Edward Arnold, 1973.

Hallowell, Nina. "Reconstructing the Body or Reconstructing the Woman? Perceptions of Prophylactic Mastectomy for Hereditary Breast Cancer Risk." In *Ideologies of Breast Cancer: Feminist Perspectives*, edited by Laura K. Potts, 153–180. New York: Palgrave Macmillan, 2000.

Hannah-Moffat, Kelly, and Pat O'Malley. "Gendered Risks: an Introduction." In *Gendered Risks*, edited by Kelly Hannah-Moffat and Pat O'Malley, 1–29. New York: Routledge-Cavendish, 2007.

Harden, Jeni. "There's No Place Like Home: The Public/Private Distinction in Children's Theorizing of Risk and Safety." *Childhood* 7 (2000): 43–59.

Harmon, Amy. "Cancer Free at 33, but Weighing a Mastectomy." *New York Times*, September 16, 2007.

Harris, Gardiner. "It Started More Than One Revolution." *New York Times*, May 30, 2010.

———. "Panel Unanimously Recommends Cervical Cancer Vaccine for Girls 11 and Up." *New York Times*, June 30, 2006.

———. "U.S. Approves Use of Vaccine for Cervical Cancer." *New York Times*, June 9, 2006.

Hart, Roderick. *Modern Rhetorical Criticism*. 2nd ed. Boston: Allyn & Beacon, 1997.

Hartmann, Lynn C., Daniel J. Schaid, John E. Woods, Thomas P. Crotty, Jeffrey L. Myers, P. G. Arnold et al., "Efficacy of Bilateral Prophylactic Mastectomy in Women with a Family History of Breast Cancer." *New England Journal of Medicine* 340 (1999): 77–84.

Hausman, Angela. "Direct-to-Consumer Advertising and Its Effect on Prescription Requests." *Journal of Advertising Research* 48 (2008): 42–56.

Hayden, Sara. "Revitalizing the Debate Between <Life> and <Choice>: The 2004 March for Women's Lives." *Communication and Critical/Cultural Studies* 6 (2009): 111–131.

"Heather Burcham on the HPV Vaccine." May 8, 2007. YouTube video. At http://www
.youtube.com/watch?v=OIsWB348z-Q. Accessed May 1, 2010.

Herskovitz, Beth. "Brand of the Year." *Pharmaceutical Executive*, February 1, 2007. At
http://pharmexec.findpharma.com/pharmexec/Articles/Brand-of-the-Year/Article
Standard/Article/detail/401664. January 22, 2012.

Himmelstein, David U., and Steffie Woolhandler. "Obama's Reform: No Cure for What
Ails Us." *British Medical Journal* 340 (2010): 742.

Hochman, David. "Mommy (And Me)." *New York Times*, January 30, 2005.

Hoffman, Jan. "A Heroine of Cocktail Moms Sobers Up." *New York Times*, August 16,
2009.

Hoover, Derrick J., Prakash R. Paragi, Elissa Santoro, Sarah Schafer, and Ronald S. Chamberlain. "Prophylactic Mastectomy in High-Risk Patients: A Practice-Based Review of
the Indications." *Breast Disease* 31 (2010): 19–27.

Horn, Suzanne M. Letter to the Editor. *Houston Chronicle*, February 12, 2007.

Houppert, Karen. "Who's Afraid of Gardasil?" *The Nation*, March 26, 2007. At http://
www.thenation.com/article/whos-afraid-gardasil. Accessed January 22, 2012.

Huckerby, Jayne. "Women Who Kill Their Children: Case Study and Conclusions Concerning the Differences in the Fall from Maternal Grace by Khoua Her and Andrea
Yates." *Duke Journal of Gender Law & Policy* 10 (2003): 150–171.

Humphries, Drew. *Crack Mothers: Pregnancy, Drugs, and the Media*. Columbus: Ohio
State University Press, 1999.

Johnson, Davi A. "Managing Mr. Monk: Control and the Politics of Madness." *Critical
Studies in Media Communication* 25 (2008): 28–47.

Johnson, Dirk, and Carol Rust. "'Who's Babysitting the Kids?'" *Newsweek*, January 17,
2005, 37.

Jordan, Julie. "She Is My Beginning." *People*, February 28, 2011, 60–66.

Katz, Alan. Letter to the Editor. *New York Times*, February 10, 2007.

Kessler, Bree, and Summer Wood. "A Shot in the Dark: What—and Who—Is Behind the
Marketing of Gardasil?" *Bitch Magazine*, Summer 2007, 27–32.

King, Samantha. *Pink Ribbons, Inc.: Breast Cancer and the Politics of Philanthropy*. Minneapolis: University of Minnesota Press, 2006.

Klawiter, Maren. *The Biopolitics of Breast Cancer: Changing Cultures of Disease and
Activism*. Minneapolis: University of Minnesota Press, 2008.

Koedt, Anne. "The Myth of the Vaginal Orgasm." In *Radical Feminism*, edited by Anne
Koedt, Ellen Levine, and Anita Rapone, 198–207. New York: Quadrangle, 1973.

Kolata, Gina. "Panel Urges Mammograms at 50, Not 40." *New York Times*, February 15,
2010.

Koopman, Cheryl, Lisa D. Butler, Catherine Classen, Janine Giese-Davis, Gary R. Morrow, Joan Westendorf, Tarit Banerjee, and David Spiegel, "Traumatic Stress Symptoms
among Women with Recently Diagnosed Primary Breast Cancer." *Journal of Traumatic
Stress* 15 (2002): 277–287.

Krishnan, Shobha S. *The HPV Vaccine Controversy. Sex, Cancer, God, and Politics: A
Guide for Parents, Women, Men, and Teenagers*. Westport, Conn.: Praeger, 2008.

Kushner, Rose. *Breast Cancer: A Personal History and Investigative Report*. New York:
Harcourt, Brace, Jovanovich, 1975.

Largo-Jannssen, Toine. "Sex, Gender and Health: Developments in Research." *European
Journal of Women's Studies* 17 (2007): 9–20.

Leopold, Ellen. *A Darker Ribbon: Breast Cancer, Women, and Their Doctors in the Twentieth Century*. Boston: Beacon Press, 1999.

Lerner, Barron H. "Inventing a Curable Disease: Historical Perspectives on Breast Cancer." In *Breast Cancer: Society Shapes an Epidemic*, edited by Anne S. Kasper and Susan J. Ferguson, 25–50. New York: St. Martin's Press, 2000.

Lerner, Sharon. "Medical Students Go Beyond Books to Learn about Activism." *New York Times*, December 2, 2003.

Lorde, Audre. *The Cancer Journals*. Special edition. San Francisco: Aunt Lute Books, 1997.

Lupton, Deborah. "Femininity, Responsibility, and the Technological Imperative." *International Journal of Health Services* 24 (1994): 73–90.

———. "Introduction: Risk and Sociocultural Theory." In *Risk and Sociocultural Theory: New Directions and Perspectives*, edited by Deborah Lupton, 1–11. Cambridge: Cambridge University Press, 1999.

———. "Risk and the Ontology of Pregnant Embodiment." In *Risk and Sociocultural Theory: New Directions and Perspectives*, edited by Deborah Lupton, 59–85. Cambridge: Cambridge University Press, 1999.

MacKeen, Dawn. "Taking the Reins on 'Gossip' and Cancer." *Los Angeles Times*, May 3, 2008.

MacLaggan, Corrie. "Health Panel Gets Testimony on Vaccine." *Austin-American Statesman*, February 20, 2007.

———. "Perry Bows to Vaccine Order's Foes." *Austin-American Statesman*, May 9, 2007.

———. "Perry Requires HPV Vaccine for Girls." *Austin-American Statesman*, February 3, 2007.

———. "Perry's HPV Vaccine Order Draws Backlash from GOP." *Austin-American Statesman*, February 6, 2007.

———. "A Push to Start HPV Shots This Fall." *Austin-American Statesman*, February 13, 2007.

Main, Kelley J., Jennifer J. Argo, and Bruce A. Huhmann. "Pharmaceutical Advertising in the USA: Information or Influence?" *International Journal of Advertising* 23 (2004): 119–142.

Mamo, Laura. "Fertility, Inc." In *Biomedicalization: Technoscience, Health, and Illness in the U.S.*, edited by Adele E. Clarke, Janet K. Shim, Laura Mamo, Jennifer Ruth Fosket, and Jennifer R. Fishman, 173–196. Durham, N.C.: Duke University Press, 2010.

Martinez, Renee, Ingrid Johnston-Robledo, Heather M. Ulsh and Joan C. Chrisler. "Singing 'the Baby Blues': A Content Analysis of Popular Press Articles about Postpartum Affective Disturbances." *Women & Health* 31 (2000): 37–56.

McElroy, Steven. "Christina Applegate Battling Cancer." *New York Times*, August 4, 2008.

McNeil, Donald G., Jr. "How a Vaccine Search Ended in Triumph." *New York Times*, August 29, 2006.

McRobbie, Angela. *The Aftermath of Feminism: Gender, Culture and Social Change*. Los Angeles: Sage, 2009.

Meijers-Heijboer, Hanne, Cecile T. M. Brekelmans, Marian Menke-Pluymers, Caroline Seynaeve, Astrid Baalbergen, Curt Burger, Ellen Crepin, Ans W. M. van den Ouweland, Bert van Geel, and Jan G. M. Klij. "Use of Genetic Testing and Prophylactic Mastectomy and Oophorectomy in Women with Breast or Ovarian Cancer from Families with a BRCA1 or BRCA2 Mutation." *Journal of Clinical Oncology* 21 (2003): 1675–1681.

"Merck Gardasil HPV Vaccine I Chose Ad #1." June 11, 2008. YouTube video. http://www.youtube.com/watch?v=ehvxbEOgNEM&feature=related. Accessed May 1, 2010.

Milford, Elizabeth Beiter. Letter to the Editor. *New York Times*, February 10, 2007.

Miller, Laura J. "Postpartum Depression." *Journal of the American Medical Association* 287 (2002): 762–765.

Modleski, Tania. *Feminism without Women: Culture and Criticism in a Postfeminist Age.* London: Routledge, 1999.

Mohanty, Chandra Talpade. "Feminism without Borders." In *Feminist Frontiers.* edited by Verta Taylor, Nancy Whittier, and Leila J. Rupp, 97–102. 8th ed. Boston: McGraw-Hill, 2009.

Mol, Annemarie. *The Logic of Care: Health and the Problem of Patient Choice.* London: Routledge, 2008.

Morgen, Sandra. *Into Our Own Hands: The Women's Health Movement in the United States, 1960–1990.* New Brunswick, N.J.: Rutgers University Press, 2002.

Murphy, Michelle. "Immodest Witnessing: The Epistemology of Vaginal Self-Examination in the U.S. Feminist Self-Help Movement." *Feminist Studies* 30 (2004): 115–147.

Myhre, Jennifer. "The Breast Cancer Movement: Seeing Beyond Consumer Activism." *Journal of the American Medical Women's Association* 54 (1999): 29–30.

Nack, Adina. "Bad Girls and Fallen Women: Chronic STD Diagnoses as Gateways to Tribal Stigma." *Symbolic Interaction* 25 (2002): 463–485.

———. "Why Men's Health Is a Feminist Issue." *Ms. Magazine*, Winter 2010. At http://www.msmagazine.com/winter2010/menshealth.asp. Accessed January 22, 2012.

Naderi, Poova S. D., and Brian D. Meyer. "Privatization within the Dutch Context: A Comparison of the Health Insurance Systems of the Netherlands and the United States." *Health* 14 (2010): 603–618.

Nelson, James. Letter to the Editor. *Austin-American Statesman*, February 9, 2007.

Nelson, Jennifer. "'All This That Has Happened to Me Shouldn't Happen to Nobody Else': Loretta Ross and the Woman of Color Reproductive Freedom Movement of the 1980s." *Journal of Women's History* 22 (2010): 136–160.

———. "'Hold Your Head Up and Stick Out Your Chin': Community Health and Women's Health in Mound Bayou, Mississippi." *National Women's Studies Association Journal* 17 (2005): 99–118.

Nicolson, Paula. "Postpartum Depression: Women's Accounts of Loss and Change." In *Situating Sadness: Women and Depression in Social Context*, edited by Janet M. Stoppard and Linda M. McMullen, 113–138. New York: New York University Press, 2003.

Nirenejca. Letter to the Editor. *USA Today*, September 6, 2008.

O'Hara, Michael W. "Postpartum Depression: What We Know." *Journal of Clinical Psychology* 65 (2009): 1258–1269.

Olesen, Virginia L., and Adele E. Clarke. "Resisting Closure, Embracing Uncertainties, Creating Agendas." In *Revisioning Women, Health, and Healing: Feminist, Cultural, and Technoscience Perspectives*, edited by Adele E. Clarke and Virginia L Olesen, 355–357. New York: Routledge, 1999.

Ono, Kent A. "Postracism: A Theory of the 'Post'- as Political Strategy." *Journal of Communication Inquiry* 34 (2010): 227–233.

Oprah Winfrey Show. Episode "Christina Applegate: Why She Had a Double Mastectomy." ABC. Broadcast September 30, 2008.

O'Reilly, Andrea. *Feminist Mothering.* New York: SUNY Press, 2008.

Palmer, Phyllis Marynick. "White Women/Black Women: The Dualism of Female Identity and Experience in the United States." *Feminist Studies* 9 (1983): 151–170.

Park, Alice. "Postpartum Depression Strikes New Fathers Too." *Time*, May 18, 2010. At http://www.time.com/time/health/article/0,8599,1989805,00.html. Accessed January 22, 2012.

Perry, Rick. "Letter Accompanying the Announcement of the Decision Regarding HB 1098." May 8, 2007. http://www.nccconline.org/health_news/topics/controversial/rick_perry.html. Accessed May 1, 2010.

———. "Gov. Rick Perry's Remarks on the Decision Regarding House Bill 1098." May 8, 2007. At http://governor.state.tx.us/news/speech/5525/. Accessed January 22, 2012.

Peterson, Alan, and Deborah Lupton. *The New Public Health: Health and Self in the Age of Risk.* London: Sage, 1996.

Pezzulo, Phaedra. "Resisting 'National Breast Cancer Awareness Month': The Rhetoric of Counterpublics and Their Cultural Performances." *Quarterly Journal of Speech* 89 (2003): 345–365.

Phillips, Alberta. "Furor Shows That What's Right Isn't Always Popular." *Austin-American Statesman*, February 26, 2007.

Philips, Anne. "Feminism and Liberalism Revisited: Has Martha Nussbaum Got It Right?" *Constellations* 8 (2001): 249–266.

Pollack, Andrew, and Stephanie Saul. "Lobbying for Vaccine to Be Halted." *New York Times*, February 21, 2007.

Polzer, Jessica, and S. Knabe. "Good Girls Do . . . Get Vaccinated: HPV, Mass Marketing and Moral Dilemmas for Sexually Active Young Women." *Journal of Epidemiology and Community Health* 63 (2009): 869–870.

Polzer, Jessica, and Ann Robertson. "From Familial Disease to 'Genetic Risk': Harnessing Women's Labour in the (Co)Production of Scientific Knowledge about Breast Cancer." In *Gendered Risks*, edited by Kelly Hannah-Moffat and Pat O'Malley, 31–55. New York: Routledge-Cavendish, 2007.

"Postpartum Depression in Men?" *The Week*, May 19, 2010. At http://theweek.com/article/index/203133/postpartum-depression-in-men. Accessed January 22, 2012.

Press, Andrea L., and Elizabeth R. Cole. *Speaking of Abortion: Television and Authority in the Lives of Women.* Chicago: University of Chicago Press, 1999.

Press, Nancy, Susan Reynolds, Linda Pinsky, Vinaya Murthy, Michael Leo, and Wylie Burke. "'That's Like Chopping off a Finger Because You're Afraid It Might Get Broken': Disease and Illness in Women's Views of Prophylactic Mastectomy." *Social Science and Medicine* 61 (2005): 1106–1117.

"Preventing Cancer or Promoting Sex?" *Dallas Morning News*, February 10, 2007.

Queller, Jessica. Interview by Renée Montagne. *Morning Edition*, National Public Radio, aired April 1, 2008.

———. *Pretty Is What Changes: Impossible Choices, the Breast Cancer Gene, and How I Defied My Destiny.* New York: Spiegel & Grau, 2008.

Rabin, Roni. "Doctor-Patient Divide on Mammograms." *New York Times*, February 15, 2010.

———. "Having a Baby: Depression Affects New Fathers, Too." *New York Times*, May 25, 2010.

———. "Health Disparities Persist for Men, and Doctors Ask Why." *New York Times*, November 14, 2006.

———. "Study Finds Rise in Choice of Double Mastectomies." *New York Times*, October 23, 2007.

Rabinow, Paul. *Essays on the Anthropology of Reason.* Princeton, N.J.: Princeton University Press, 1996.

Railsback, Celeste Condit. "The Contemporary American Abortion Controversy: Stages in the Argument" [1984]. In *Readings on the Rhetoric of Social Protest*, 2nd ed., edited by

Charles E. Morris III and Stephen Howard Browne, 472–485. State College, Pa.: Strata Publishing, 2006.

Reinhardt, Uwe E., Peter S. Hussey, and Gerard F. Anderson. "U.S. Health Care Spending in an International Context." *Health Affairs* 23 (2004): 10–25.

Rich, Adrienne. "Compulsory Heterosexuality and Lesbian Existence." In *The Lesbian and Gay Studies Reader*, edited by Henry Abelove, Michele Aina Barale, and David M. Halperin, 227–254. New York: Routledge, 1993.

———. *Of Woman Born: Motherhood as Experience and Institution.* 1986; repr., New York: Norton, 1995.

Roberts, Lynn. "March to Save Women's Lives." *Collective Voices* 1 (2003): 4.

Robertson, Ann. "Embodying Risk, Embodying Political Rationality: Women's Accounts of Risks for Breast Cancer." *Health, Risk, and Society* 2 (2000): 219–235.

Rose, Nikolas. "Beyond Medicalization." *The Lancet* 369 (2007): 700–702.

———. *The Politics of Life Itself: Biomedicine, Power, and Subjectivity in the Twenty-first Century.* Princeton, N.J.: Princeton University Press, 2006.

———. *Inventing Our Selves: Psychology, Power and Personhood.* Cambridge: Cambridge University Press, 1996.

———. "Will Biomedicine Transform Society? The Political, Economic, Social and Personal Impact of Medical Advances in the Twenty First Century." *BIOS Working Papers* (2008): 3–20. At http://www.crassh.cam.ac.uk/uploads/documents/Rose%20N.pdf. Accessed February 23, 2012.

Rosser, Sue V. "An Overview of Women's Health in the U.S. Since the Mid-1960s." *History and Technology* 18 (2002): 355–369.

Rothman, David J., and Sheila M. Rothman. "Marketing HPV Vaccine: Implications for Adolescent Health and Medical Professionalism." *Journal of the American Medical Association* 302 (2009): 781–786.

Ruzek, Sheryl Burt, and Julie Becker. "The Women's Health Movement in the United States: From Grass-Roots Activism to Professional Agendas." *Journal of the American Medical Women's Association* 54 (1999): 4–8.

Saporito, Bill. "He Won His Battle with Cancer. So Why Are Millions of Americans Still Losing Theirs?" *Time*, September 15, 2008, 36–42.

Sardenberg, Cecilia M. B. "Liberal vs. Liberating Empowerment: A Latin American Feminist Perspective on Conceptualising Women's Empowerment." *IDS Bulletin* 39 (2008): 18–27.

Saul, Stephanie, and Andrew Pollack. "Furor on Rush to Require Vaccine." *New York Times*, February 17, 2007.

Schaffer, Amanda. "Why Are Mastectomies on the Rise?" *DoubleX*, June 17, 2009. At http://www.doublex.com/section/health-science/why-are-mastectomies-rise. Accessed January 22, 2012.

Schwartzberg, Joel. "Slouching Toward Fatherhood." *Newsweek*, April 13, 2009, 17.

Seaman, Barbara. *The Doctor's Case Against the Pill.* New York: Peter H. Wyden, 1969.

Segal, Judy. "Breast Cancer Narratives as Public Rhetoric: Genre Itself and the Maintenance of Ignorance." *Linguistics and the Human Sciences* 3 (2007): 3–23.

Shapiro, Ester. "Because Words Are Not Enough: Latina Re-Visionings of Transnational Collaborations Using Health Promotion for Gender Justice and Social Change." In *Diversity and Women's Health*, edited by Sue V. Rosser, 64–94. Baltimore, Md.: Johns Hopkins University Press, 2009.

Shelley, Donna. "Establishing Women's Health Centers in Academic Institutions: Obstacles and Opportunities." *Journal of the American Medical Women's Association* 54 (1999): 9–14.

Shen, Eveline. "Asian Communities for Reproductive Justice Answers the Question: What Is Reproductive Justice?" *Collective Voices* 1 (2004): 6.

Shields, Brooke. *Down Came the Rain: My Journey Through Postpartum Depression.* New York: Hyperion, 2005.

———. "War of Words." *New York Times,* July 1, 2005.

Siegel, Reva B. "Dignity and the Politics of Protection: Abortion Restrictions under *Casey/Carhart.*" *Yale Law Journal* 1694 (2008): 1694–1800.

Siers-Poisson, Judith. "Research, Develop, and Sell, Sell, Sell: Part Two in a Series on the Politics and PR of Cervical Cancer." *PRWatch,* June 30, 2007. At http://prwatch.org/node/6208. Accessed January 22, 2012.

Silliman, Jael, Marlene Gerber Fried, Loretta Ross, and Elena R. Gutierrez. *Undivided Rights: Women of Color Unionize for Reproductive Justice.* Cambridge, Mass.: South End Press, 2004.

Smith, Andrea. "Beyond Pro-Choice Versus Pro-Life: Women of Color and Reproductive Justice." *Feminist Formations* 17 (2005): 119–140.

Span, Paula. "Making Sure Mothers Start on the Right Foot." *New York Times,* April 9, 2006.

Springen, Karen. "No Guarantees." *Newsweek* (web exclusive), August 27, 2008. At http://www.newsweek.com/id/155864/. Accessed January 22, 2012.

Stacey, Judith. "Sexism by a Subtler Name? Postindustrial Conditions and Postfeminist Consciousness in the Silicon Valley." In *Gendered Domains: Rethinking Public and Private in Women's History: Essays from the Seventh Berkshire Conference on the History of Women,* edited by Dorothy O. Helly and Susan M. Reverby, 322–338. Ithaca, N.Y.: Cornell University Press, 1993.

Stanek, Jill. "Debbie Does . . . ??" *Illinois Review,* February 6, 2007. At http://illinois review.typepad.com/illinoisreview/2007/02/debbie_halvorso.html. Accessed January 22, 2012.

Starfield, Barbara. "Is US Health Really the Best in the World?" *Journal of the American Medical Association* 284 (2000): 483–485.

Steinem, Gloria. "Supremacy Crimes." *Ms. Magazine,* August 1999, 45.

Szabo, Liz. "Dad's Pregnancy Hormones." *USA Today,* June 15, 2010.

———. "New Dads Hit by Depression as Often as Moms." *USA Today,* May 19, 2010.

Tait, Sue. "Television and the Domestication of Cosmetic Surgery." *Feminist Media Studies* 7 (2007): 119–135.

Tarkan, Laurie. "After the Adoption, a New Child and the Blues." *New York Times,* April 25, 2006.

Tasker, Yvonne, and Diane Negra. "Introduction: Feminist Politics and Postfeminist Culture." In *Interrogating Postfeminism: Gender and the Politics of Popular Culture,* edited by Yvonne Tasker and Diane Negra, 1–26. Durham, N.C.: Duke University Press, 2007.

Taylor, Verta. *Rock-a-By Baby: Feminism, Self-Help and Postpartum Depression.* London: Routledge, 1996.

Thomasson, Melissa A. "From Sickness to Health: The Twentieth-Century Development of U.S. Health Insurance." *Explorations in Economic History* 39 (2002): 233–253.

Thompson, Marie. "Who's Guarding What? A Poststructural Feminist Analysis of Gardasil Discourses." *Health Communication* 25 (2010): 119–130.

Tolman, Deborah L. *Dilemmas of Desire: Teenage Girls Talk about Sexuality.* Cambridge, Mass.: Harvard University Press, 2002.

Tomes, Nancy. "Patient Empowerment and the Dilemmas of Late-Modern Medicalization." *The Lancet* 369 (2007): 698–700.

Traiger, Lisa. "Stomp the Stage: Tradition Meets Contemporary Rhythm at Step Afrika's Spirited Performance." *Dance Magazine*, February 2009, 40–42.

Treichler, Paula. *How to Have Theory in an Epidemic: Cultural Chronicles of AIDS.* Durham, N.C.: Duke University Press, 1999.

Tuana, Nancy. "The Speculum of Ignorance: The Women's Health Movement and Epistemologies of Ignorance." *Hypatia* 21 (2006): 1–19.

Umansky, Lauri. *Motherhood Reconceived: Feminism and the Legacy of the Sixties.* New York: New York University Press, 1996.

Vavrus, Mary Douglas. "Opting Out Moms in the News: Selling New Traditionalism in the New Millennium." *Feminist Media Studies* 7 (2007): 47–63.

———. *Postfeminist News: Political Women in Media Culture.* Albany: SUNY Press, 2002.

Vorhaus, Dan. "Breaking: District Court Rules Myriad Breast Cancer Patents Invalid." *Genomics Law Report*, March 29, 2010. At http://www.genomicslawreport.com/index .php/2010/03/29/breaking-district-court-rules-myriad-breast-cancer-patents-invalid/. Accessed January 22, 2012.

Wagman, Diana. Review of *Pretty Is What Changes*, by Jessica Queller. *Los Angeles Times*, April 27, 2008.

Weber, Lynn, and Deborah Parra-Medina. "Intersectionality and Women's Health: Charting a Path to Eliminating Health Disparities." *Advances in Gender Research* 7 (2003): 181–230.

Weiner, Lynn Y. "Maternalism as a Paradigm: Defining the Issues." *Journal of Women's History* 5 (1993): 96–130.

Weir, Richard. "Names, Dignity and Hope: Dumped, Dead Newborns Get TLC from Foundation." *New York Daily News*, March 4, 2007.

"Woman Not Guilty in Retrial in the Deaths of Her 5 Children." *New York Times*, July 27, 2006.

Wood, William C. "Editorial: More Answers About Prophylactic Mastectomy." *Annals of Surgical Oncology* 14 (2007): 3283–3284.

Yabroff, Jennie. "The Deepest Cut." *Newsweek* (web exclusive), April 14, 2008. At http:// www.newsweek.com/id/131985. Accessed January 22, 2012.

Zimm, Angela, and Justin Blum. "Merck Promotes Cervical Cancer Shot by Publicizing Viral Cause." *Bloomberg*, May 26, 2006. At http://www.bloomberg.com/apps/ news?pid=newsarchive&sid=amVj.y3Eynz8&refer=us. Accessed January 22, 2012.

Index

ACS. *See* American Cancer Society
Affordable Care Act, 163–164, 187–188
American Cancer Society (ACS), 35, 39,
 40–44
Applegate, Christina, 11, 33, 34, 46, 47, 49–
 53, 63, 64; and contralateral prophylactic
 mastectomy, 44–45, 50; and fertility, 55–
 58, 150–151; and reconstructive surgery,
 59–62
Armstrong, Heather, 71, 76, 77, 82–84, 86–
 87, 90–91, 104

BCA. *See* Breast Cancer Action
biomedical empowerment, 64–65
biomedicalization era, 14, 21, 36, 39, 65,
 109, 140, 154–155, 163
biomedicine: critiques of, 17, 142, 147, 157–
 159, 161; women's relationship with, 31,
 35, 38, 54, 64–65, 89, 140, 151–152, 177,
 183, 188
biosocial communities, 156, 161
birth control pill, 15, 16, 17, 18, 40,
 144–146
Boston Women's Health Book Collective,
 16, 19
breast cancer, 6, 10, 11, 20, 21, 26, 65–67,
 73, 87, 146, 148, 150, 172, 176, 185;
 and BRCA gene mutations, 11, 34, 39,
 41–42, 44–50, 52–58, 60, 63, 66, 86, 150,
 156, 161; and Breast Cancer Action, 37,
 66–67, 154, 157–161, 175, 177, 180, 181;
 and breast reconstruction, 61–62; chemoprevention of, 43; and chemotherapy,
 38, 46, 50, 51, 55, 67; culture, 35–40,
 42, 48, 63, 64, 67, 181; depoliticization
 of, 152–153; and mammograms, 34, 36,
 37, 38–39, 43, 48, 58, 67, 158; and the
 "one-step" procedure, 18; previvors of,
 42–44, 161; and radical mastectomy, 15,
 35, 36, 67; and risk (*see under* risk discourse); survivors, 5, 37, 39, 42, 64, 154;
 and Toxic Links Coalition, 153–154; and

visibility, 33–34. *See also* prophylactic
 mastectomy
Breast Cancer Action (BCA), 37, 66–67, 154,
 157–161, 175, 177, 180, 181; and "Think
 Before You Pink," 159–160
Burcham, Heather, 127–128, 139

Cade, Toni, 18
Casper, Monica, 107, 110
Carpenter, Laura, 107, 110
cervical cancer, 11, 26, 109–112, 125, 135,
 139–141, 148, 149, 150, 151, 152, 153;
 and the "at-risk/risky woman," 11, 108,
 135, 140, 148, 149, 151, 153; and health
 disparities, 107, 109–111, 120, 122–
 123, 149, 162, 165; medical empowerment in relationship to, 12, 108, 117,
 138–140, 152; and pap smears, 110,
 111, 132, 141, 149; and postfeminism
 (*see under* postfeminism); and postracial discourse, 114–116, 118, 120,
 122–125, 130, 131; and risk discourse
 (*see under* risk discourse); and the
 risk of sex, 108, 125, 128–134; and the
 role of daughters, 109, 115–116, 119,
 122–128, 134–135, 137–139, 142; and
 the role of mothers, 114–116, 118–
 119, 125–128, 130, 136–139, 150; and
 sexuality, 107–108, 111–112, 119, 121,
 128–132, 135–136, 138, 140–141, 153.
 See also Gardasil; HPV
Clarke, Adele, 3, 14, 22, 36, 143, 158, 177
Clarke, Juanne Nancarrow, 4
compulsory heterosexuality, 125, 171
Condit, Celeste, 166
Connors, Catherine, 80–81
consumption as empowerment, 8, 23, 54,
 116, 117, 140, 141, 153, 159
Corinna, Heather, 173–175, 179, 186. *See
 also* Scarleteen
Cruise, Tom, 86
cult of true womanhood, 125

Dean, Mitchell, 27
DES (diethylstilbestrol), 146
Douglas, Susan, 70, 99
Duggan, Lisa, 147

Eckman, Anne K., 20–22
Ehrenreich, Barbara, 87
Epstein, Stephen, 14, 19, 21–22, 146, 165,
    171–172

Facing Our Risk of Cancer Empowered
    (FORCE), 42, 49, 51, 156, 161
Fields, Jessica, 130
Focus on the Family, 129, 130, 153
FORCE. See Facing Our Risk of Cancer
    Empowered
Fosket, Jennifer, 38, 40–41, 43

Gardasil, 7, 11, 107–109, 112–113, 135, 149,
    152, 153, 185; and class privilege, 115–
    117, 136; and the Gardasil girl, 113–118,
    120–122, 124–125, 127, 128, 131, 135–
    136, 138, 149, 181; and the Gardasil girl
    narrative (see under narrative); and HPV
    risk, 112–113, 116, 119; and the "I Chose"
    campaign, 135–139; mandates, 11, 107–
    109, 121, 122–124, 126–128, 129–136,
    149, 153; and the "One Less" campaign,
    113–121, 122, 124, 127, 131, 135–137,
    139; and postfeminism (see under post-
    feminism). See also cervical cancer; HPV
genetic susceptibility, 39, 42, 62, 73, 152,
    155, 156, 178. See also breast cancer:
    BRCA gene mutations
Gessen, Masha, 48, 50, 56
Gilman, Charlotte Perkins, 72
"Go Red for Women," 1, 2, 4, 8–9, 20, 22, 23

Hall, Stuart, 3
Hallowell, Nina, 61, 62
Halverson, Debbie, 133
Hayden, Sara, 167
health care reform, 163–164, 187
health disparities, 11, 58, 109, 122–123, 149–
    150, 162–163, 170; and health inequali-
    ties, 12, 162, 165, 169–170, 171, 174, 175,
    176, 178, 188; intersectional perspective
    on, 12, 165–166, 169–170, 174

health insurance, 58, 66, 123, 162–164
heart disease, 1, 2, 4, 9, 10, 20, 21. See also
    "Go Red for Women"
heterosexual matrix, 25, 65, 128, 140–141, 171
HPV (human papillomavirus), 85, 107, 108,
    109, 120, 121, 122, 124, 137–140, 149,
    185; as common, 116, 119, 178; and fertil-
    ity, 127–128, 150; and sexual politics,
    111–113, 116–117, 119, 129–135, 141,
    153; vaccine, 110, 111, 112, 121, 124,
    126, 127, 131, 141, 149, 153. See also
    cervical cancer; Gardasil

inclusion-and-difference paradigm, 10, 21,
    22, 146, 164–165, 171, 177

Johnson, Davi, 87, 89

King, Samantha, 38
Klawiter, Maren, 35–37, 39, 48, 64, 66
Komen for the Cure, 37–38, 40–44, 147, 156
Kushner, Rose, 18, 37

Lorde, Audre, 37, 63
Lupton, Deborah, 28, 29–30, 34, 39, 133

March for Women's Lives, 167–169, 180,
    184
McRobbie, Angela, 24–26
medicalization, 14–15, 72, 75–76, 82, 85,
    87, 88, 100–101, 151, 185
medicalization era, 10, 14, 154
men's health, 1, 185
Merck, 107, 108, 112–113, 119–121, 123,
    135, 136, 138, 153
Michaels, Meredith, 70, 99
molecular gaze, 74, 85
mommy blogs, 71, 76–78, 83
motherhood, 11, 28, 55, 57, 63, 69, 76, 127,
    148, 151, 172, 181; and bad mommies,
    77–79, 91; cultural expectations about,
    28, 63, 70, 72, 74–75, 78; and feminism,
    15, 69–71, 103, 181; and the myth of the
    good mother, 70–71, 77–79, 84, 101; and
    postfeminism (see under postfeminism).
    See also postpartum depression
Myriad Genetic Laboratories, 39, 66–67

narrative, 2, 4–8, 23, 70, 82, 144, 153, 171,
178; Gardasil girl, 113–114, 116, 120,
121, 131, 135, 149; proliferation of, 12,
143, 153, 176–178, 181, 183; prophylactic mastectomy, 11, 34–35, 44–47, 49, 51,
52, 54–55, 57–58, 59–66, 99, 151, 152; of
risky motherhood, 11, 71, 77–81, 83–84,
88, 91, 92, 94, 95–96, 99–100, 102–103;
women's health, 3, 5–8, 12, 24, 32, 143,
144, 148, 161, 170–171, 178, 181, 188;
and women's identities, 2–3, 5–8, 10, 24,
35, 62, 64, 65, 71, 79, 99, 114, 116, 121,
125, 149, 153, 171, 176–177
National Black Women's Health Project, 16,
17, 168
National Cancer Institute (NCI), 40–42
National Women's Health Network, 16, 147,
152, 168
NCI. *See* National Cancer Institute
Negra, Diane, 22, 56, 58, 62
neoliberalism, 7, 9, 30, 54, 64, 89, 118, 141,
180, 181; and choice, 23, 26, 40, 117, 140,
142, 150, 153, 166–167; and economic
arrangements, 25–26, 27, 147; and health,
3, 8, 23, 24, 27, 142, 147–148, 153, 154,
171, 176, 188; and individualism, 23, 24,
31, 62, 100–101; and postfeminism (*see
under* postfeminism); and risk, 9, 41, 42,
62, 155.
Nicolson, Paula, 74

Olesen, Virginia, 143, 158, 177

Paltrow, Gwyneth, 89–90
paternalism, 3, 37, 108–109, 121–122, 124–
125, 126, 128, 135
Perry, Rick, 107, 108, 121, 123, 126, 127,
139; and arguments for vaccine mandate,
122, 124, 129, 132–133
Peterson, Alan, 28, 29, 39, 133
Pezzullo, Phaedra, 153–154
Polzer, Jessica, 31, 120, 176
postfeminism, 9, 10, 13, 22–26, 148–153;
and body modification, 23, 54, 59, 62; and
cervical cancer, 108–109, 124, 128, 140,
149, 153; and choice, 12, 13, 23, 30, 32,
34, 49, 54–55, 80, 108, 116, 117, 124, 136,
139–140; and class privilege, 3, 35, 45,

58, 80, 99, 101, 115, 148–149, 167–168,
170; and consumption, 23, 54, 125, 140,
141, 147, 159; and femininity, 10, 23–25,
59; and Gardasil, 113, 114, 116, 117–118,
125, 128, 131, 136, 139, 149, 153; and
girl power, 116, 118; and individualism,
23–24, 27, 55, 100, 124, 152, 161, 180;
masquerade, 24–25; and motherhood, 76,
80–82, 84, 92, 94–95, 99, 100–101, 103;
and neoliberalism, 3, 7, 8, 9, 23–24, 54,
64, 100–101, 140, 142, 148, 153, 171, 176,
181; and postpartum depression, 81, 82,
84, 92, 95, 99, 100–101, 103, 151; and
prophylactic mastectomies, 34–35, 45, 49,
54, 55, 57, 58–59, 62, 63, 64, 66, 150; and
race privilege, 3, 35, 45, 58, 80, 99, 101,
114, 148–149, 167–168, 170; and risk (*see
under* risk discourse); and traditional gender roles, 10, 24, 55, 57, 63, 81, 109, 140,
142, 150, 171, 178; and the vulnerable
empowered woman (*see under* vulnerable
empowered woman); and women's health,
3, 7, 8, 10, 12, 13, 22, 23, 24, 26–27, 32,
66, 99, 141, 143, 145, 147–148, 150–153,
155, 159, 161, 168, 169, 170, 171, 176,
181, 183
postpartum depression, 7, 11, 71–76,
102–103, 148, 150, 151–152, 153, 162,
172, 181; and adoptive parents, 105; and
class, 101–102, 162; destigmatization of,
75, 84, 85–87, 151; and empowerment,
91–94, 98, 99–100, 102; and fathers, 94,
103–105; and feminism, 72, 74–75, 103,
151, 181; and hormones, 73, 76, 85–86,
103–105, 152; and love of children,
79, 81, 88; medicalization of, 72, 75,
85–88, 100, 101, 151; and the monstrous
mother, 94, 96–98, 101; and the narrative of risky motherhood (*see under*
narrative); normalization of, 71, 81, 82–
83, 87, 88, 92, 97, 99, 101, 151; and postfeminism (*see under* postfeminism); and
race, 101–102, 162; and recovery, 82, 91,
94, 98; risks associated with (*see under*
risk discourse); and the risky mother,
71, 81, 83–89, 91–94, 97, 99–102, 103,
150; and self-discipline, 89, 91, 100;
and self-help, 37, 45, 75, 103, 151;

postpartum depression (*continued*)
and self-surveillance, 89–93, 98, 101,
102; social context as explanation for,
72, 74–76, 103–105, 151, 181; and surveillance, 92–94, 99–102, 151; symptoms of, 71, 73, 82, 87, 88, 94; treatment
of, 86, 93–94, 97–98

Postpartum Progress blog, 85, 86, 91, 94, 96

postpartum psychosis, 71, 72, 73, 95–96, 98,
101, 102, 151

prophylactic mastectomy, 5, 7, 11, 43–45,
63–65, 80, 99, 142, 150–151, 152; and the
cancer/risk-free woman, 10, 11, 35, 44,
45, 52–53, 58–59, 62, 63–65, 148, 150,
151, 152, 153, 176; as choice, 11, 34, 44,
49, 52–58, 63, 150; and family and fertility, 34–35, 44, 46, 55–58, 60, 63, 150–151;
and femininity, 59–61; and narrative (*see
under* narrative); and postfeminism (*see
under* postfeminism); and privilege, 35,
58–59, 62, 64–65; and reconstructive
surgery, 59–62; as refusal of cancer risk,
45–46, 51–53, 63, 64. *See also* breast
cancer

Queller, Jessica, 11, 34, 44–61, 63, 64, 150

Reach for Recovery, 36, 63
representational politics, 5, 65
reproductive health, 165–167
reproductive rights, 19, 146, 167, 169, 188
rhetorical criticism, 8
Rich, Adrienne, 69, 71, 125
risk discourse, 24, 27–32, 129, 151, 153,
155, 172; and breast cancer, 35, 36, 39–
44, 45–50, 52–54, 57, 62–63, 64, 66, 151,
156, 161, 176, 180; and cervical cancer,
108, 111, 114–115, 116–117, 119–120,
121, 125, 129–130, 140, 141; and health,
10, 28–32; and heart disease, 8–9; and
postfeminism, 13, 27, 30, 57, 178; and
postpartum depression, 80–81, 86, 88–89,
91, 95, 99, 97, 101, 104; and pregnancy,
30, 172

Robertson, Ann, 10, 31, 176

Rose, Nikolas, 14, 18, 39, 41–42, 65, 75, 100,
141, 152, 154, 155–157

Ross, Loretta, 17, 168, 169

Scarleteen, 173–175, 177, 178–181

Seaman, Barbara, 145, 147

Segal, Judy, 6

sex education, 130, 173–174. *See also*
Scarleteen

sexually transmitted infections and/or diseases, 107, 111, 117, 120, 121, 123, 130,
135, 138, 153, 166; and stigma, 112–113;
and youth, 119, 132, 134, 173, 178–179.
See also HPV

Shields, Brooke, 71, 76–77, 79, 85–87,
89, 90, 95, 96, 97, 101; surveillance of,
92–93, 99; and symptoms of postpartum
depression, 82–83

SisterSong Women of Color Reproductive
Justice Collective, 168–169, 175, 180, 181

Smith, Andrea, 166

sterilization abuse, 15, 17

Tasker, Yvonne, 22, 56, 58, 62

Taylor, Verta, 72, 74, 103

traditional womanhood, 24, 26, 27, 35, 55,
124, 172

Tuana, Nancy, 16

Vavrus, Mary Douglas, 82, 148, 188

vulnerable empowered woman, 3, 8–10,
47, 63, 88, 135, 148, 151–153, 177; and
postfeminism, 9, 24, 26, 35, 151, 180,
183; and the reification of gender roles, 9,
24, 26; revisioning of, 178–181

war on cancer, 33

Women in Government, 107, 135, 153

women's health: and biomedicine, 147, 148,
151–152, 158–159, 183; and biosocial communities, 156–157, 161; depoliticization of,
3, 9, 21, 152–153, 183; and elite/privileged
women, 3, 7, 17, 19, 80, 148–149, 162,
168, 170; and empowerment, 2, 8, 24, 32,
54, 141, 148; and feminism, 8, 10, 13–19,
22–23, 37, 66, 72, 88, 146–147, 153, 176,
181, 185–186, 188; and gender roles, 3, 24,
26, 150, 171–176, 183; and narratives (*see
under* narrative); and a new feminist health
politics, 143, 153–176, 177–178, 181; and
postfeminism (*see under* postfeminism);
proliferating narratives about, 176–177;

visibility of, 1, 2, 7, 8, 9, 20, 146–147, 153.
See also women's health movement
Women's Health Initiative, 20
women's health movement, 10, 13–22, 55,
    144–145, 146, 154, 176–177, 185; critical
    stance of, 2, 122, 147; epistemology and,
16–17, 157; feminist perspective of, 2, 8,
15, 19; self-determination and, 17–18, 54;
race and, 14, 16, 18–19

Yates, Andrea, 71, 96–98
Yentl Syndrome, 20–21

About the Author

Tasha N. Dubriwny is an assistant professor in the Department of Communication and the Women's and Gender Studies Program at Texas A&M University. She has published essays on women, health, and politics in *The Quarterly Journal of Speech*, *Women's Studies in Communication*, and *The Journal of Communication Inquiry*.

Available titles in the Critical Issues in Health and Medicine series:

Emily K. Abel, *Suffering in the Land of Sunshine: A Los Angeles Illness Narrative*

Emily K. Abel, *Tuberculosis and the Politics of Exclusion: A History of Public Health and Migration to Los Angeles*

Marilyn Aguirre-Molina, Luisa N. Borrell, and William Vega, eds. *Health Issues in Latino Males: A Social and Structural Approach*

Susan M. Chambré, *Fighting for Our Lives: New York's AIDS Community and the Politics of Disease*

James Colgrove, Gerald Markowitz, and David Rosner, eds., *The Contested Boundaries of American Public Health*

Cynthia A. Connolly, *Saving Sickly Children: The Tuberculosis Preventorium in American Life, 1909–1970*

Tasha N. Dubriwny, *The Vulnerable Empowered Woman: Feminism, Postfeminism, and Women's Health*

Edward J. Eckenfels, *Doctors Serving People: Restoring Humanism to Medicine through Student Community Service*

Julie Fairman, *Making Room in the Clinic: Nurse Practitioners and the Evolution of Modern Health Care*

Jill A. Fisher, *Medical Research for Hire: The Political Economy of Pharmaceutical Clinical Trials*

Alyshia Gálvez, *Patient Citizens, Immigrant Mothers: Mexican Women, Public Prenatal Care and the Birth Weight Paradox*

Gerald N. Grob and Howard H. Goldman, *The Dilemma of Federal Mental Health Policy: Radical Reform or Incremental Change?*

Gerald N. Grob and Allan V. Horwitz, *Diagnosis, Therapy, and Evidence: Conundrums in Modern American Medicine*

Rachel Grob, *Testing Baby: The Transformation of Newborn Screening, Parenting, and Policymaking*

Mark A. Hall and Sara Rosenbaum, eds., *The Health Care "Safety Net" in a Post-Reform World*

Beatrix Hoffman, Nancy Tomes, Rachel N. Grob, and Mark Schlesinger, eds., *Patients as Policy Actors*

Laura D. Hirshbein, *American Melancholy: Constructions of Depression in the Twentieth Century*

Timothy Hoff, *Practice under Pressure: Primary Care Physicians and Their Medicine in the Twenty-first Century*

Rebecca M. Kluchin, *Fit to Be Tied: Sterilization and Reproductive Rights in America, 1950–1980*

Jennifer Lisa Koslow, *Cultivating Health: Los Angeles Women and Public Health Reform*

Bonnie Lefkowitz, *Community Health Centers: A Movement and the People Who Made It Happen*

Ellen Leopold, *Under the Radar: Cancer and the Cold War*

Barbara L. Ley, *From Pink to Green: Disease Prevention and the Environmental Breast Cancer Movement*

David Mechanic, *The Truth about Health Care: Why Reform Is Not Working in America*

Alyssa Picard, *Making the American Mouth: Dentists and Public Health in the Twentieth Century*

Heather Munro Prescott, *The Morning After: A History of Emergency Contraception in the United States*

David G. Schuster, *Neurasthenic Nation: America's Search for Health, Happiness, and Comfort, 1869–1920*

Karen Seccombe and Kim A. Hoffman, *Just Don't Get Sick: Access to Health Care in the Aftermath of Welfare Reform*

Leo B. Slater, *War and Disease: Biomedical Research on Malaria in the Twentieth Century*

Paige Hall Smith, Bernice L. Hausman, and Miriam Labbok, *Beyond Health, Beyond Choice: Breastfeeding Constraints and Realities*

Matthew Smith, *An Alternative History of Hyperactivity: Food Additives and the Feingold Diet*

Rosemary A. Stevens, Charles E. Rosenberg, and Lawton R. Burns, eds., *History and Health Policy in the United States: Putting the Past Back In*

Barbra Mann Wall, *American Catholic Hospitals: A Century of Changing Markets and Missions*

DATE DUE

PRINTED IN U.S.A.

CPSIA information can be obtained at www.ICGtesting.com
Printed in the USA
BVOW030021031012

301889BV00003B/3/P

9 780813 554006